RETURNING T

GW00391045

IPLINARY LIBRARY

ON
SUhPE
on or before the last d

RETURNING TO NURSING

A Guide for Nurses and Health Visitors

Alison Morton-Cooper, RGN

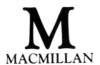

MACMILLAN

REDHILL MULTIDISCIPLINARY LIBRARY
REDHILL HOSPITAL
EARLSWOOD COMMON
REDHILL, SURREY.

© Alison Morton-Cooper 1989

All rights reserved. No reproduction, copy or transmission
of this publication may be made without written permission.

No paragraph of this publication may be reproduced, copied
or transmitted save with written permission or in accordance
with the provisions of the Copyright Act 1956 (as amended),
or under the terms of any licence permitting limited copying
issued by the Copyright Licensing Agency, 33–4 Alfred Place,
London WC1E 7DP.

Any person who does any unauthorised act in relation to
this publication may be liable to criminal prosecution and
civil claims for damages.

First published 1989

Published by
MACMILLAN EDUCATION LTD
Houndmills, Basingstoke, Hampshire RG21 2XS
and London
Companies and representatives
throughout the world

Typeset by Footnote Graphics, Warminster, Wilts
Printed in Great Britain by
Camelot Press Ltd, Southampton

British Library Cataloguing in Publication Data
Morton-Cooper, Alison
Returning to nursing.
1. Medicine. Nursing – Manuals
I. Title
610.73
ISBN 0–333–48076–7

5226

WY16

Robinson 12/90.
£5.95

RSH

To Dad, for believing in miracles

Contents

Acknowledgements   viii
How to Use This Book   ix
Foreword   xi

Introduction   1

1   Deciding to Return   3

2   Building Professional Confidence   19

3   Practical Issues at Home and Work   37

**4   The Back to Nursing Movement and Prospective
     Employers**   49

5   The NHS and its Mid-life Crisis   81

6   Returning to Learning   101

7   Changes in Nursing Practice   117

Postscript   133

Appendix 1   The UKCC Code of Professional Conduct
     for the Nurse, Midwife and Health Visitor   134
Appendix 2   Nursing Journals Available from High Street
     Newsagents   136
Appendix 3   Careers Information Addresses   138
Index   139

Acknowledgements

I would like to extend my sincere thanks to the many nurses, nurse tutors and health visitors who have assisted me in the preparation of this book by responding to my requests for advice with enthusiasm and generosity.

They include: Marilyn Castle, labour relations officer, Royal College of Nursing; Shirley Goodwin, general secretary of the Health Visitors' Association; Peta Allan, director for professional standards and development at the UK Central Council for Nursing, Midwifery and Health Visiting; Reg Pyne, director for professional conduct at the UKCC; the chief executives of the four National Boards: Lyn Mitchell, David Ravey, J. Walsh and David Jones; Mrs Jean Heath of the ENB Careers Advisory Service; Martin Vousden of *Nursing Times*.

I owe a great deal to the patience and forbearance of my editorial board, Frances Pickersgill, Philip Burnard, and Tony O'Malley, and to my publisher Mary Waltham for inspired leadership. The book could not have been completed without the assistance of Ann Banfill, or the encouragement of my husband Barrie, and of my son, Alastair, who has learned the secret of playing to the whirr of the typewriter.

AMC, June 1989

How to Use This Book

Returning to Nursing is aimed at all qualified nurses and health visitors hoping to return to practice after a career break.

Written with the aspirations and concerns of returners in mind, it provides a re-introduction and update on many of the issues already encountered by experienced nurses, and an introduction to new concepts and developments in line with current recommendations and guidelines on preparation for re-entry.

In the extensive research undertaken for the book it became clear that a number of particular issues posed the greatest challenges to potential returners and to prospective employers. The chapters which follow therefore address these directly. By raising the awareness of returning nurses and health visitors of such important issues as professional accountability, new approaches to the learning process and the learning environment, the implications of research based care and the impact of new technologies in nursing, I hope that the book will help to facilitate a safe and knowledgeable return to practice for both the individual returner and her employer.

The book may be used by individuals or as a companion text to Back to Nursing programmes. Chapters 2 and 7 particularly are intended to provoke discussion and debate, and to provide a basis for independent and group study as seminar or project work before, or in conjunction with, supervised clinical allocations.

Selective annotated bibliographies address clinical and professional topics ranging from individualised care planning to drug administration, safe handling skills, wound management, the nurse's role in cardiopulmonary resuscitation and many other more specialised skills.

The book is very much a general introduction, aimed at providing nurses of all specialties with the essential practical background information required to negotiate a successful return to practice.

Popular nursing mythologies are demystified and explained and advice given on tailoring re-entry preparation to suit individual learning needs. By concentrating on the practical implications of new ideas this book should help to promote positive strategies for welcoming nurses and health visitors back to practice at a time when their skills are needed and sought after as never before in the profession's long and distinguished history.

Foreword

Tomorrow, today will be the 'good old days'. It is easy to make lasting judgements based on impressions and recollections from a time when things were different. It is a fact of our lives that change is constant and that change is often feared. It is also very easy to lose touch. Following a break in nursing practice there may be an understandable hesitation and anxiety about returning because of the inevitable changes that will have taken place. There is also an anxiety that through losing touch with developments, skills are also lost. Circumstances such as these can lead to real apprehension about returning to practice.

This book is a practical and timely guide to the journey leading to that return. It chronicles recent changes within the professions and the health services and is a useful source of reference and information. It is written in a reassuring way that should positively assist nurses, midwives and health visitors and allay understandable anxieties.

The context in which care is given is also subject to change as, indeed, are the professions themselves. Organisational arrangements, educational systems and approaches to treatment and care are all in a continuing state of change and development. For the professions to be sensitive to change, and to meet the needs of patients and clients there must be a constant readiness to develop and adjust to accommodate new challenges. Changes in practice, in turn, call for changes in education and in the professions to ensure that the needs of society are met effectively and that standards are safeguarded for our patients and clients.

The professions, collectively, must face these challenges. Individuals returning to practice also face a personal challenge and have their own needs for support and encouragement so that their important transition from a break to return to practice is assisted. This book should assist this process and help practitioners focus on what personal qualities and skills they bring and not just those areas in which help and information may be required. The personal and life experiences which all practitioners bring to practice can enrich nursing, midwifery and health visiting teams and, in turn, the care they give.

I hope that this book will be a major source of practical advice and assistance and will encourage the return of practitioners.

Colin Ralph
Registrar and Chief Executive
United Kingdom Central Council for
Nursing, Midwifery and Health Visiting

Introduction

The importance of managing a career break effectively is now widely recognised. New initiatives aimed at attracting nurses back to work are springing up and developing throughout the UK. Service managers are waking up to the value of experienced nurses whose understandable reservations about being out of date with current ideas and technologies prevent them from taking up their careers again.

At the moment it is theoretically possible for a qualified nurse with 20 years' break in service to be put in charge of an acute ward, and to take responsibility for the management and allocation of staff, even though she may not have any recent or relevant experience. This is clearly undesirable for the nurse, the staff, and most of all the patient, who has a right to expect expert care and attention.

The statutory bodies for nursing, midwifery and health visiting have functions clearly defined in law which are concerned with ensuring proper standards of care. Proposals to introduce mandatory re-entry programmes for nurses and health visitors linked to periodic relicensing are one way of maintaining a safe level of practice, and a logical step forward in promoting the importance of maintaining such safety.

The central policy-making body for the professions, the United Kingdom Central Council for Nursing, Midwifery and Health Visiting (UKCC), has already issued guidelines for good practice[1] aimed at improving the standard and content of re-entry programmes available to qualified nurses and health visitors wishing to update their clinical and theoretical knowledge.

This book uses as its framework and *raison d'être* the concept of mandatory re-entry programmes for nurses and health visitors with a break in practice of five years or more, as put forward by the UKCC in 1989.

The lack of one central source of information and guidance on the provision of programmes, and on the process of re-entry, can make attempts to return something of an exercise of faith and perseverance.

This book is designed to help you cut out the hard work, and instead redirect your energies into formulating a worthwhile, personally relevant and practical route into the kind of nursing which appeals to you or suits you best at this particular stage in your career.

Reference

1. *Guidelines for Good Practice: return to practice programmes for nurses and health visitors*, document PS and D/86/06 (London: UKCC, 1986).

CHAPTER 1

Deciding to Return

Making the decision to resume a demanding job or career is a serious and sometimes hazardous business; not least because it requires a thorough review and reappraisal of your lifestyle.

If you are single and ambitious, then your career pattern and development will be important to you, and any prospects for promotion in the longer term are a significant factor when looking for the right opening. If you are married, or committed to a serious relationship, have one child or more and a home to support, then the hours you work and the amount of travel involved in getting to and from work may limit your options.

I have been careful not to make any assumptions about you. I have avoided attempting to stereotype you and the life you lead. From my own experience of listening to nurses who want to return, the reasons they give and the levels of motivation they express are multifarious. It may be that the untapped pool of non-practising nurses are in the main housewives and mothers, or frustrated office workers. If you are either, or both, and you feel that your time has come, then there is much relevant information for you in the chapters ahead.

The men and women I have met come from all sorts of social and employment backgrounds. Some have reluctantly had to give up an earlier nursing career because of ill health, or to care for a dependent partner, close relative or friend. Frequent house moves caused by a partner's promotion may have made any long-term employment unviable. Some have worked abroad as volunteers, on extended vacations or in casual jobs, and have then found it difficult to get back into the mainstream of a career. Others who have been in permanent employment as

3

nurses have found the restrictions of poor pay and stringent working conditions too harsh.

As a result, they have been forced into less desirable but more lucrative employment elsewhere in order to support an 'acceptable' standard of living. Often softened by nostalgia for what they recall as the security of their 'training days', I have heard older nurses enthuse about the cosiness and order of day to day nursing. Distant recollections of established routines and clearly defined duties represent a world where the ability and willingness to carry out instructions was of paramount importance.

Bridging the gap

As a general nurse who trained in a large London teaching hospital, and qualified shortly before the demise of the General Nursing Councils and the introduction of the new statutory bodies for nursing, midwifery and health visiting, I have found listening to the reminiscences of those who have experienced a considerable career gap both salutary and frightening. Salutary, because I am made more aware of the advances made in developing the nursing role in health care. Frightening, because the apparent chasm stretching from past to present experience seems vast and commands respect.

The challenges facing nurses in the 1990s are likely to be as great as any the profession has ever faced. No one could or should pretend that nursing in the future will resemble nursing in the past.

If you are fortunate enough to live in an area where the local district health authority (DHA) has a positive and dynamic recruitment policy, then bridging the gap between jobs will be high on its list of priorities. If it already runs a back to nursing course then it will also have established a policy geared towards attracting you back to work. The types of courses available are looked at in detail in chapter 4.

If you should decide to accept a place on a course, do not rush out to buy textbooks until you have finished reading this book, and guidance on returning to learning in particular. Lengthy booklists are expensive and dull: with some time and effort it will be possible for you to build up a personal library and reference system which is individually geared to your particular needs, and one which helps you to build on your existing knowledge rather than attempting to start again from scratch.

If for some reason you cannot or choose not to attend a course, then you will have to find some means of charting your progress with the limited help made available by colleagues. If you live or work within borrowing distance of a nurse education centre, then you should ask for the name of the post-basic or continuing education tutor. Even if he or she does not answer to this title directly, there is usually one member of staff who has responsibility for supporting and assisting qualified staff with their continued professional education. The nursing and medical libraries can be made accessible to you, as can the skills of the librarian, for whom finding that elusive reference you have searched for can become a personal crusade.

Reviewing career goals

Detecting and quantifying the innate personal attributes of the effective nurse has puzzled recruiters for many years. Recent attempts by psychologists to arrive at psychological tests which identify desirable characteristics in candidates has had only limited success. The criteria for selection which rest on school examination results and rapport with the interviewer are still widely used. Mature students who lack the requisite O-levels or GCSEs can opt to sit an alternative entrance test, although there is some confusion over the purpose of such tests. Are they designed to assess levels of intellectual ability, or do they have an ulterior motive in seeking to shine a light on a suitable psyche? Who knows what makes a good nurse? Definitions often dry on the tongue.

Nursing has been described as a skilled occupation rather than a profession. You will either belong and adhere to this school of thought, or you will be outraged at the very suggestion. A skilled occupation is a more accurate description of the task-oriented kind of care carried out by tradition. As the eminent nursing historian Monica E. Baly points out, in the nineteenth century sense nursing did not qualify for pro-

5

fessional status: '... nurses were not independent practitioners and indeed, the insistence on obedience was anti-ethical to independence and self-sufficiency'.[1]

I assume therefore, that Monica Baly's own definition of a profession rests at least in part on independence and self-sufficiency. Professionalism implies a contract with society; a promise that good faith will be justified. If you trust to a lawyer or a doctor, then it will be against his code of ethics to betray that trust. In her book *Professional Accountability*, Monica Baly takes this a stage further:

> If professions have an implied contract with society which gives them 'status, authority and privilege' then society wants certain assurances in return ... skill is not enough, there must be a code of ethics which indicates how clients and patients should be served and the attitudes that should be accepted ... Clearly, no one should enter a profession without subscribing to its fundamental tenets.

Perhaps the most important and far-reaching change in nursing in the past ten years has been the wholesale move away from the subservient, passive role of the nurse who was accountable to doctors for any treatments she undertook, and to nursing supervisors for standards of personal conduct and discipline.

The emphasis placed on current practice could be described as self-sufficiency; an ability to make and act upon decisions arrived at from a position of sound professional judgement, decisions arrived at independently of doctors but complementary to their assessment of patients. Doctors are expected to assess medical needs; nurses are themselves expert at assessing nursing need, or to put it another way, at assessing the need for nursing aspects of care.

In choosing to nurse, you therefore must take on board the ethics required of your chosen profession. These have now been laid down by the UKCC in its *Code of Professional Conduct for the Nurse, Midwife and Health Visitor*.[2]

The introduction to the code is crystal clear:

> Each registered nurse, midwife and health visitor shall act, at all times, in such a manner as to justify public trust and confidence, to uphold and enhance the good standing and reputation of the

profession, to serve the interests of society, and above all to safeguard the interests of individual patients and clients.

The code goes on to outline what is required of a registered practitioner in the exercise of 'professional accountability'. A closer examination of the component parts of the code is given in chapter 4, when we begin to look at the implications of the code in respect of standards of nursing care provided by the qualified nurse or health visitor.

How you measure up to making decisions in the light of your clinical and theoretical knowledge will have a direct bearing on the quality of care you are able to give. The ability to assess, plan, implement and evaluate care, whatever your area of clinical expertise, will become a large part of your role as a qualified nurse.

Nursing need not necessarily be viewed as a career. I have heard many other definitions (not all of them polite), but most people agree that advancement of some sort features in their long-term plans for the future.

Proposed changes in the clinical career structure should make clinical nursing less of a poor relation in terms of financial recognition and status. The old standards of nursing management having superior status to clinical nurses are gradually phasing themselves out, and certainly in the future you will not have to move away from the bedside solely to boost levels of pay.

When reviewing your own goals for the future, it might be useful to look at some of the positive aspects of nursing as a career, to see whether you still identify with them.

Nursing can provide me with:

● An opportunity to work with and care for people of all races, communities and creeds.
● The satisfaction of helping fellow human beings in need.
● Work which is relevant to family life, where skills acquired may be utilised outside the immediate work environment.
● A wide variety of specialisms which can be adapted to suit my own interests and aptitudes.
● Opportunities for promotion once I have made a clear commitment to the work.

7

- Work which will enable me to travel abroad.
- Work which can earn me money in my spare time.
- Work which can be used as a stepping stone to another career.

If reforms in the career structure and nursing education go ahead as planned, then you may be able to add the following to your list:

- More realistic pay, dependent on my level of expertise and the amount of responsibility I hold
- An environment in which the nursing student is supernumerary, with improved facilities for teaching and for sharing my teaching role with other colleagues.
- Opportunities for the development of clinical and managerial skills, with a clearer role for the specialist nurse practitioner and adviser.

If you want to go back to basics and try to assess the sort of person you are, and the kind of working environment best suited to you, then there are a number of exercises you can do with an honest friend. These are explained in Jill Baker's book *What Next?* If you lack this insight or are looking for a new direction, then Baker can help (see Recommended reading at the end of this chapter).

Most of you, however, will already have a good idea of where you would feel most secure. This may be your principal guide in choosing a route of re-entry. If the reason you left nursing in the first place was boredom or disillusionment, it may be that you had drifted into an environment which failed to take advantage of your best qualities.

If so, now is the time to decide exactly what it was that made the work so stale and uninteresting. Consider the following, and see how many words or phrases describe your feelings – as you remember them – at the time you left nursing.

- Bored
- Frustrated
- Undervalued
- Lacking in confidence

- Scared of making a mistake
- Confused or unsettled
- Keen, but thwarted by managers
- Overmanaged
- Professionally isolated
- Impatient for results

If any of the first five are included in your list, take heart, because these can be dealt with and are avoidable. The second five are more difficult, but probably say a great deal about the style of management you worked under, and the quality of relationships you had with colleagues and peers. It is also important to look at why you took up the job in the first instance, even if 20 years have elapsed in the meantime. This might have coloured your attitude to the work, and be relevant when you want to make a fresh start:

- It was the only vacancy offered to me at the time
- The hours suited me
- I desperately wanted to work there
- I was told it would be 'good experience' for me
- I do not really remember
- I liked the staff running the ward/unit
- I enjoyed the specialty
- I was marking time until something better came along

More than two negative reasons for accepting a job can take a heavy toll on your resources of enthusiasm, particularly if you had the added disappointment of being turned down for the post you'd really hoped for at the time.

Assessing your motivation to return

Having made a tentative decision to come back to nursing, it would be similarly useful to compare your reasons for doing so in the light of the previous exercise.

Are you bored with your present job? Is this your only alternative to unemployment? Have you missed nursing and long to return? You may know of someone who has already tried it and succeeded. You may be attracted by an advertise-

9

ment in your local paper, or perhaps reading the nursing press has aroused your interest. Perhaps your domestic circumstances have changed, and you are now able to resume what was once an enjoyable way of earning a living. You may feel guilty at letting hard-won skills go to waste. You may have heard very positive things about a local employer. You may, dare I say it, need the money.

It can be quite illuminating to write down a few vague goals, and then to discover just how deepseated your real feelings about nursing can be. If you can do this after an informal interview or visit then so much the better. One glimpse of a resuscitation trolley or a bunch of keys can be enough to send any romantics back to their Mills & Boon!

Motivation may be nine tenths necessity. The vital tenth, an enthusiasm for the work itself, is a helpful prerequisite, especially when it comes to convincing a prospective employer. He or she will want to be convinced that you are serious in intent, and will also want to be reassured of your staying power. The costs involved in properly re-orientating and updating staff are considerable. The argument that this is money well spent only bears out if you then follow up with a reasonable period of reliable service.

Opinions vary as to what constitutes 'reasonable' in this case. If you are put in the position of having to commit yourself to one employer, establish well in advance of accepting a job or secondment offer exactly what will be required of you in terms of subsequent employment. If you have decided to train for an entirely new specialty, such as health visiting or district nursing, you may find yourself having to reimburse course and equipment fees if you leave the job before a specified date of up to two years after your training has been completed. If this seems unreasonable to you, you may want to reconsider.

Nursing in the marketplace

Your skills are in short supply and have acquired a rarity value undreamed of in the 1970s. One visit to a nursing careers fair will convince you of this. The shortage is worldwide.

Selling your skills

This may sound a rather aggressive and mercenary way to go about things, but it is the philosophy to which I am referring, rather than your personal approach. I do not expect you to haggle, for example, but an element of bartering over hours and conditions can improve your working life considerably. What employers will be interested in is the confidence and faith you have in yourself to revise and update your clinical skills in order to place them in a service context.

Before putting yourself or your past experience down, as too many nurses are inclined to do, think instead about the stressful situations and important decisions you have had to face since leaving nursing. If you have brought up a family, and survived, then you are more than capable for anything nursing can throw at you. Do not underestimate the value of life experience; that is your natural instinct and ability to overcome whatever obstacles or hindrances are put in your way.

So many returners admit to stage fright at the beginning of a re-entry programme, only to find that the expectations of managers and colleagues are much more realistic than they have given them credit for. It is far from the interests of your employer to scare you into a kind of beavering submission.

Employers will, of course, want to make clear to you the level of personal responsibility you will be expected to take within the remit of your job description (for a sample job description, see chapter 2), but this doesn't necessarily mean that they are trying to warn off the less confident. It is you they need, and your skills they must be prepared to help you to adapt and improve. I am not going to suggest that you play hard to get. You never know who is behind you in the queue. What I am suggesting is that you should not underrate your ability to succeed in what is now a highly competitive market place.

Acquiring new skills

The lazy among us will always claim that it is more difficult to learn as you get older. This is a matter of fierce debate. A willingness to learn and perseverance are much more important than candles on a birthday cake. Much really depends on the quality of opportunities open to you to refresh old skills, and to introduce new ones on a sensible timescale and with proper supervision and support. You will not have to depend on now or never clinical demonstrations in the clinical room; nor will you be reduced to knock-kneed terror at the prospect of a *viva voce* examination. The education of nurses is now much more student-centred, focusing on the consolidation of skills already mastered, and on the gradual introduction of new and unfamiliar techniques by practice and experience.

Your personal experience of relationships and interaction with others can be enhanced and built upon in a constructive way, thus helping to inspire both personal confidence and a learning environment where you will not be inhibited from admitting to a lack of knowledge or understanding. Passive acceptance and rote learning of facts and procedures is now discouraged; you will instead be expected to participate fully in an exchange of views and information. At the same time you will have the benefit of your supervisor's own competence and expertise on the subject.

All this could come as a shock to your system if you were the shy and reticent student who hid behind more extrovert colleagues. The reassurance that there is a place for all of us in the scheme of things should help a little. The virtual extinction of the dragon sister tutor should also help to allay your fears.

The UKCC Code of Professional Conduct states that every nurse, midwife or health visitor should 'Take every reasonable opportunity to maintain and improve professional knowledge and competence'. This includes the acquisition of any new and relevant skills and applies equally to staff employed on a full or part-time basis; in the public and the private sector. This means that you have a responsibility to find 'reasonable opportunities' by actively seeking them. Make clear to your new employer that you are looking forward to continuing your professional education. They should be well placed to help you to help yourself.

You may find that after an initial burst of enthusiasm, your employers run out of steam and seem reluctant to fund you on courses or give you conference or study leave. Ironically, it is sometimes shortage of staff which prevents them from letting you go. Until you and other recruits swell the establishment figures, pressure on service managers will continue.

Occasionally politics comes into this, and you may notice that the same member of staff always gets the best deal. Be prepared to question this if you want to, and do not retreat from any withering looks. Even if you work only a small number of hours, you still need to review and assess your progress on a regular basis. Any opportunity to advance your studies should be seen as an important part of your continuing in-service education.

Expanding opportunities in the NHS, the private sector and abroad

As the available range of therapies and treatments grows, there is no doubt that opportunities for in-depth specialisation in supporting patients or clients grow with it. Rigid divisions of patients by medical condition are much less usual now, and remain the province of obsessional medical students and old school consultants, for whom classification by organ is a time-honoured tradition.

The number and variety of specialties open to qualified nurses is wide, and probably has no equal in any other profession. If your plan is to move ahead quickly and gain promotion in as short a time as possible, you would probably fare best in an area where the shortage of suitably qualified staff is most acute. To be taken seriously, you will have to demonstrate an understanding of the problems facing the specialty you want to work in, and be able to communicate sound ideas for progress. Qualities of leadership and innovation are always in short supply. It is no accident that men fill most of the top jobs in nursing, while women remain on the lower grades.

The reorganised NHS will – for most of you – be the first port of call when looking for new employment. It may be that you feel most secure in returning to a familiar environment. For all but a few of you, however, the pattern of working and the hierarchy itself will have changed beyond recognition. It is certainly true that the priorities favoured by one style of management have no guarantee of being upheld by another.

A move from consensus management, where a small, but arguably representative nucleus of people had at least some say in the decision-making, to a more dictatorial style known as 'general management' now means that decisions are made by one man or woman who may accept or reject the advice of interested parties, including nursing and medical advisers.

The idea, introduced by Sainsbury's chairman Sir Roy Griffiths in his 1983 review of NHS management, is vested in meeting business-like objectives, with stricter costing of the service, and unit managers being held directly responsible for staying within set targets and providing an adequate service at the same time.

As part of your readjustment you will find yourself becoming much more cost conscious, and aware of the cost implications of continuing with practices which may be wasteful, or unwieldy, given cheaper alternatives. One of the most striking examples of this is the policy on drug prescription. More generic drugs are now used, and stocks are much more carefully controlled. Likewise sterile supplies and instruments are less plentiful than you may remember. Different units will have found different ways of saving money. This is a potential source of conflict between service staff and managers if the service side feel that supplies are inadequate or to the detriment of patients.

Regardless of your area of specialisation, the old epithet of 'tried and trusted' has been replaced by experimentation and sometimes cursory evaluation of what is achieved by one approach to a nursing procedure over another. On the positive side, high quality nursing research has begun to have an effect on the way nursing practice is carried out. The importance of knowing why we do things and not just what to do has altered many of the concepts and shattered many long held perceptions about the effectiveness and quality of care we give to patients. An appreciation of the whys and wherefores of nursing research is fundamental to good practice and an introduction to this for the uninitiated appears in chapter 7.

It is change of this kind which is more likely to surprise and challenge you when you first return.

If you should decide to concentrate on one particular nursing specialty then you will probably want to undertake a clinical nursing studies course. The Joint Board for Clinical Nursing Studies disappeared in 1983 when the new statutory bodies for nursing came into existence. The work of the JBCNS, the General Nursing Councils, the Central Midwives' Boards, the Council for the Education and Training of Health Visitors, the

Committee for Clinical Nursing Studies and the Panel of Assessors for District Nurse Training was taken over by the new United Kingdom Central Council and four National Boards for England, Scotland, Wales and Northern Ireland, respectively. Although the UKCC is the central policy making and administrative body responsible for setting and maintaining professional standards, and much more (see chapter 5), it is the national board of the country in which you choose to practice that is responsible for executive action on nurse education, ensuring that it meets the UKCC's rules and requirements.

Postbasic certificate and statemented (the latter are generally shorter) courses are validated by the boards and a list of current courses and training establishments can be obtained by writing directly to the boards or to a delegated careers advice service. Useful addresses appear in the Appendices.

You can also enquire locally to see whether your local DHA has details of course vacancies. Different centres of excellence will usually offer courses in their own specialism; you may find you have to work away from home on secondment if your first choice is limited to only a few specialist centres. Examples of this are courses in accident and emergency, neuromedical and neurosurgical nursing or ophthalmic nursing.

The trend in nursing education certainly favours the progression of clinical nursing specialists. If you are interested in the current thinking on this the RCN has recently published a useful document *Specialities in Nursing*.[4]

Public or private sector employment?

Your chances of promotion to a position of responsibility in nursing and health visiting are undoubtedly greater in the NHS, if only because of its number of employees. As the largest public sector employer in Europe it can offer scope for experience in management and education, in research and in clinical nursing itself. However, there are many new avenues opening up for qualified staff in areas which have not traditionally been associated with nursing. Joint initiatives between establishments of higher education and health authorities offer a more dynamic and interdisciplinary approach to learning, with virtually unlimited scope for a career in lecturing, research or publishing.

Entrepreneurial skills are also being utilised, with more nurses going into business for themselves; running employment agencies, nursing homes and conference organisations. The independent sector continues to grow, particularly in the fields of routine and day surgery and health screening.

Health visitors are rarely employed as such outside the NHS, although the qualification itself can provide an entry gate to other positions, particularly in advisory capacities to child health and other voluntary organisations, in health education and teaching at tertiary and higher education levels. Health visitors who study for a further education teacher's certificate can be employed as curriculum planners and lecturers on nursery nursing courses and pre-vocational courses aimed at recruitment to the NHS.

The view that private sector employment is a waste of valuable career time is less widely held, now that the private sector is beginning to take its share of providing additional training and in-service education facilities for its own employees. In some cases joint ventures between the private sector and the NHS are succeeding in taking on areas which are proving too costly or cumbersome for the NHS alone.

Ideologically you may be committed to working for the NHS. This should pose no problems. If you are in a quandary, however, as to which to choose, and are unsure of the different kinds of work available in both sectors, you could begin by reading the classified advertisements in either *Nursing Times* or *Nursing Standard*. Both carry details of jobs in the independent sector and the *Standard* has occasional recruitment supplements which may look in more depth at job opportunities. You could also try working for a nursing agency. This way you may be able to get a taste of different or unusual working environments before committing yourself to one or the other. Some agencies are particularly keen to attract nurses who have had a break in practice and provide reorientation for new staff. Agency nursing and the option of working in a nurse bank run by NHS or private hospitals is discussed in more detail in the next chapter.

Nursing abroad

The lure of glossy full colour advertising, particularly when it depicts sparkling blue skies, golden beaches, and smiling, sun-kissed offduty nurses, is potent and seductive.

But, however confident you are after being wooed and won by an overseas recruiter, you may feel isolated and vulnerable once you have signed a contract and find that you are on your own. If you are seriously contemplating taking your˙ skills abroad, then it may be advisable to invest some time in updating yourself at home first. If you are uncomfortable with the idea of attending a local NHS run course, then some form of distance learning package, which involves studying at home with some tutorial support, may be what you need to get you started.

It is also wise to seek the advice of the international department of your professional organisation. The RCN runs a comprehensive advisory service for its members and can offer the benefit of continued professional indemnity insurance.

Attempting to take up a post abroad without any preparatory updating could be courting disaster. If your new employer has offered to provide you with facilities for updating, make sure that this is included in your contract of employment, and that it is backed up with meaningful support and supervision. You do not want to run the appreciable risk of making a bad mistake before your new career has really started.

References

1.   M. E. Baly, *Professional Responsibility* (Chichester: John Wiley & Sons, 1984).
2.   UKCC, *Code of Professional Conduct for the Nurse, Midwife, and Health Visitor*, 2nd edn (London: UKCC, 1984).
3.   R. Griffiths, *NHS Management Inquiry Report* (London: DHSS, 1983).
4.   RCN, *Specialities in Nursing* (Harrow: Scutari Projects Ltd, 1988).

Recommended reading

J. Baker, *What Next? Postbasic Opportunities for Nurses* (Basingstoke: Macmillan Education, 1988).
M. E. Baly, *Professional Responsibility* (Chichester: John Wiley & Sons, 1984).

CHAPTER 2

Building Professional Confidence

Reassessing your skills

According to McEvoy[1] self-evaluation is the hallmark of the reflective practitioner. Certainly some reliable measure of the way you deliver nursing care is necessary and valuable, both for the client (or patient) and his environment, and ultimately for the sense of satisfaction you can enjoy yourself as a reflective practitioner of nursing.

As McEvoy suggests, time, like money, should be budgeted: 'The reflective practitioner will avoid taking on more than he or she can accomplish calmly and effectively ... If nurses were as careful with time as they tend to be with money, their professional effectiveness would take a meteoric rise'.

Your personal recollection of evaluation may be limited to semi-formal evaluation 'sessions' tacked onto the end of a study block or course, when you were invited to give your personal views and answer preset questions on the strengths and weaknesses of the work or study methods, quality of lectures, usefulness of discussions and so on. Nowadays evaluation has a tendency to be much more structured and less prosaic.

Self-evaluation requires you to be completely honest with yourself, but in a constructive rather than a negative way. You may be dissatisfied with your reflection in the mirror but you do have to admit that it has its good points! In the same way, self-evaluation can mirror those things which require reappraisal, those which only require a little attention, and those which need a complete overhaul. Reassessing the skills you bring back to nursing or health visiting can be a worthwhile preparation for returning to practice, even if you feel a poor judge of what skills might be most needed in the future.

Judging by the experience of former returning nurses it is the professed loss of practical and handling skills which gives rise to most worry. It does not help when tutors attempt to compare such skills to riding a bicycle. Perhaps you were always a bit wobbly anyway! You may have recollections of taking a long time to achieve competence in one particular skill, and wonder whether on returning you will be given adequate time to practise and revise.

If you had anticipated returning to clinical nursing without undertaking a re-entry programme first, then this kind of worry will have to be ironed out during your period of reorientation to the ward or district. If you are in this position, or even if you are lucky enough to have obtained a place on a re-entry course, it may help to make a tentative assessment of the skills you feel need to be reassessed in order to practise safely.

Identifying your learning needs

Sooner or later you will be given an opportunity to discuss your learning needs with a senior nurse. This may be a tutor, ward sister or charge nurse, or a member of the ward team who is designated to work as a 'mentor' – a personal counsellor and guide throughout your reorientation period and even beyond. As a starting point, try drawing up individual lists of skills, dividing them into:

● Those you could do straight away.
● Those you feel you would soon revise and become competent in.
● Those you would feel unhappy about attempting without first having received advice and instruction.

This can be a useful group exercise as well as an individual one. If you are going to confide in each other, however, it is important to respect each other's different tolerance levels. Some people can feel very intimidated and experience a temporary crisis of confidence, especially if they have been in employment which is entirely unrelated to nursing. Years away from the bedside can distort your view.

Past experience in nursing can also reflect a very hierarchical, even military approach, and some 'procedures' may have suffered at the hands of obsessional and aggressive teaching. Fortunately, much more than rote learning of 'trays, trolleys and treatments' is now expected, and a preoccupation with rigid routines is a thing of the past.

Once you have completed the basic exercise given above you will have a ready reference on which to draw when identifying your personal learning needs. It helps if you can limit your first list to those skills you will require in one clinical area. In this way you will not be overwhelmed by too many gaps and can build on your experience one stage at a time.

Acknowledging your limitations

Even if there are significant gaps in your knowledge it should be possible to get help with these in advance of being given clinical responsibility.

One problem which has been described to me by nurses and health visitors who returned to practice before the advent of re-entry programmes is the difficulty represented by assumed knowledge. The depth of knowledge assumed by colleagues who have never experienced a break in service can undermine the confidence of returners, even if the supposed lack of knowledge is more imagined than real.

Admitting to a lack of knowledge or competence is embarrassing and difficult, particularly if time and staff are limited and something needs to be done quickly. Identifying these areas is not always easy or straightforward. They cannot always be anticipated. You may not realise until you are asked that you do not have the skills required.

The UKCC Code of Professional Conduct[2] (see Appendix 1, clause 4) is very clear in stating your obligation here:

Acknowledge any limitations of competence and refuse in such cases to accept delegated functions without first having received instruction in regard to those functions and having been assessed as competent.

Failure to take due regard of this obligation places your patients at risk and may jeopardise your right to practise. Your position could not be clearer.

Of course life is not always as simple as that, and being asked to cover for a colleague at very short notice or an unexpected cancellation or transfer on the theatre list can throw your best laid plans into disarray.

When discussing the lessons, problems and failures arising from the disciplinary hearings of the former General Nursing Councils, Reg Pyne, now the UKCC's director for professional conduct, extends this obligation to nurse managers[3]:

> Nurse managers have a responsibility for the settings in which patients are cared for which is far greater than the same responsibility of nurses at large, simply because they are employed in positions which enable them to make appropriate representations. They bear this responsibility not only that the patients may receive safe and competent nursing care but that the nurses working in those settings are not rendered vulnerable by excessive pressure.

Not only is it unprofessional to fail to acknowledge your limitations, it is equally unprofessional for managers to delegate care to a nurse who is unsure of her ability to implement it safely.

However, this still does not tell you what to do in a crisis or if an unexpected emergency arises.

If you are unfortunate enough to be faced with such a situation then the only responsible advice I can suggest is the same as that offered to nursing students. Refuse. Refuse politely, out of earshot of the patient involved, and give your reasons why. Regardless of the experience of your senior nurse momentary aberrations do occur, particularly under pressure, and he or she may simply not have realised the implications of what was being asked.

I can think of very few occasions when you would not have the time to state your case. If the situation is one of life or death, and you are the only person available, then it could be argued that you should not deny whatever limited skills you have to the person whose life is in danger. This is a grey area which depends a great deal on the actual situation, and it may be worthwhile introducing it to discussions with managers or teachers for the benefit of other nurses, and to share ideas on how you would approach such a problem.

Self help

Most employers are only too keen to introduce new employees gently to their employment. It is difficult for them to know just how great are the gaps in your knowledge and the limitations on your competence, and so they will depend on you to make your own initial assessment.

Any learning process is a continuum dependent on listening, hearing, observing, questioning, listening, hearing, observing and then understanding. Breaks in this chain can inhibit the learning process and lead to a breakdown in effective communication.

Listening to yourself can be a first step in identifying a learning need or goal.

- I don't know enough about . . .
- My concentration is poor.
- I can't digest this information.
- I don't understand why this should happen.
- I get the two things confused.

Try writing down those things which you feel you absolutely need to know more about before being given responsibility. This differs from the previous exercise in that you are not looking directly at skills, but at the theoretical knowledge you require to undertake those skills safely. I run the risk of sounding patronising here, but I do feel that this is a point worth making.

You may be surprised at the length and diversity of this list. You may find that a pattern emerges, or that one subject or area comes up time and time again.

To take this a stage further I would like to paraphrase the skills outlined in a sample job description, and identify some learning needs which might arise from it. If you have already been offered a job and have agreed on a job description with your future service manager, then you may like to analyse it in the same way.

'The staff nurse, in the absence of the ward sister or charge nurse shall:
● Lead and co-ordinate ... to ensure that the programme of each patient's care ... is effective and meets the individual patient's needs.
● Assume responsibility for teaching and supervising all (nursing) team members.'
'As part of everyday responsibilities she shall:
● Interpret the significance of clinical observations and records, making appropriate decisions, and planning nursing care accordingly.
● Assist in delegated clinical research.
● Determine nursing priorities on a daily basis and plan patient care according to staff availability and capabilities.
● Maintain an awareness of circumstances which can affect standards of care and act accordingly.
● Inform and support relatives as appropriate.
● Maintain professional confidentiality.
● Ensure accuracy and legibility of clinical and legal documents.
● Encourage good working relationships and communication networks within the health care team.
● Ensure continuity of care.'

The above is only an extract from a full job description but nevertheless I can already identify four areas where I would need guidance and information before I would feel capable of meeting my responsibilities safely.

1 Teaching skills, as appropriate to the particular clinical setting and those I am expected to teach.
2 Clinical research skills. Having no real experience of clinical research I would need to undertake some form of assisted learning in research appreciation and the application of practical research skills.
3 Management skills. These may need to be reviewed and updated in line with my new clinical environment, and a new or different approach to team management.

4 I would need to revise my knowledge of patient/client confidentiality so that I may not inadvertently be in breach of proper professional conduct.

This exercise should help to clarify the kind of theoretical and practical knowledge you need to update and give you valuable insight into the nature of the job before you return to practice safely and enjoyably.

Job expectations and rewards

Expectation and reward are entirely subjective, and a matter of personal preference. Your expectations of future employment will be influenced by your past experience and any feedback you have had more recently from people in similar jobs.

Watson discusses the meaning of work[4] and separates motivation to work into intrinsic and extrinsic satisfactions. Human groups may vary as to the extent they are able to gain satisfaction of either type:

Examples of intrinsic satisfactions

● Inherent satisfaction
● Personal fulfilment.
● Something to take a pride in.
● An increase in self-esteem.
● Work which is enriching.

Examples of extrinsic satisfactions

● I oing the work for financial gain.
● Needing 'the company' of others in the work team or setting.
● Work used as a means to an end.

Watson[4] stresses the importance of the individual's personality as a factor influencing the meaning and value of work on a personal level, but adds that additional factors such as age, upbringing, sex, education, nature of employing organisation and social class matter too. From a sociologist's point of view, work has shades of meaning which are individual to each of us. Nursing as work or as a vocation can mean different things to different people.

Presumably most of us work for the same principal reason – in order to live – but the choice of job may be influenced more by necessity than choice. Options available may be severely limited by matters of health, geographical location, intelligence, family commitments and job availability. What attracts a nurse or health visitor back to practice is likely to be a combination of intrinsic and extrinsic factors. Historically, nursing has probably offered a mix of both satisfactions, although financial gain would probably come quite a way down on the list.

The general public has a tendency to assume that nurses experience a strong desire to care for others, perhaps believing that many feel a true vocation or 'divine call' to the work, although it is probably less usual to describe it in these terms today. Because aspects of the work are those which are less palatable to some, being considered as messy or 'dirty' work, there is an implied element of personal sacrifice and supplication on behalf of those who are sick and perhaps suffering.

Professor Chapman[5] breaks down potential nurses into two distinct categories. The first is prepared to accept certain personal sacrifices in order to care for others; the second is the frustrated medic – the nurse who ideally would be studying medicine or one of the biological sciences. The latter is more likely to seek work in such areas as intensive care or renal dialysis where equipment is likely to be intricate and of vital importance, rather than in those areas requiring mainly basic physical care of the patient. Professor Chapman[5] points out that this does not necessarily lead to a drop in standards of physical care, but stresses the apparent risk that patients may occasionally be made to feel 'merely an appendage to a machine'.

A natural consequence of an affinity to mechanical things, and an ability, what is more, to master them, is generally accorded more status than direct patient contact. Such jobs enjoy a higher status and may be considered more popular and glamorous than others. As Professor Chapman observes, high status nursing can be seen as a route to social mobility; the more closely the nurse works with a doctor as a member of the team, the more prestigious the job is assumed to be.

If your expectations or primary motivation in doing a particular job is to be upwardly mobile, it is unlikely that you are going to want to get involved in a job which remains at the bedside. Recent trends in the professions have, however, challenged this way of thinking. Both professional organisations and the statutory bodies have worked hard to achieve a career structure which rewards so-called 'hands on' nursing, and moves away from a system whereby the standard route for promotion is removal from direct patient care into a separate hierarchical management role.

Financial rewards

Attempts to restructure and remunerate accordingly are the basis of the new clinical grading exercise introduced in 1988. By assessing each post individually, the peculiar responsibilities of the post will be identified and the nurse placed on a pay scale which recognises her experience and expertise. The regrading of every qualified nurse in post has of course proved to be a colossal and traumatic exercise for both management (acting under Department of Health directives) and the nursing unions whose job it is to mediate on behalf of members.

It is the level of the government's ongoing commitment to honour the recommendations over pay and conditions of the Nurses' and Midwives' Pay Review Body (PRB) which has so incensed the professions. The sometimes insensitive and arbitrary methods employed in carrying out the regrading exercise has aroused scorn, derision and even despair from those who were led to believe that substantial pay increases were to be honoured at last. By October 1988, the original deadline for the completion of the regrading exercise, both the unions and management had still to reach agreement.

Although the government had set aside over £800 million to cover regrading and the funding of the 1988 pay award, additional pressures were being put on DHAs to find the money for any shortfall in their budgets from their service budgets. The implication of moral blackmail in robbing patient services to pay nurses remained a ghost at the banquet for the media, and for many nurses, who had still to reconcile the jobs they had perhaps been doing for years with the management's idea of

27

their responsibilities, and the clinical grade to which they aspired.

It would be worthless to dwell on the strengths and weaknesses of the regrading exercise here, other than to acknowledge the apparent difficulties associated with it. In the context of nurses and health visitors returning to work it might be more useful to look at the ways in which regrading affects your application and appointment, and to provide you with general advice on what to expect from employers in due course.

Clinical grading and the returner

Table 2.1 is general advice, obtained from the Labour Relations department of the RCN. Any specific queries arising from it may be addressed to your local branch steward if you have one. Members of the Confederation of Health Service Employees (COHSE) and the National Union of Public Employees (NUPE) should also approach their stewards for help. Contact names and numbers can usually be found on staff noticeboards or obtained from regional offices. Members of the HVA can contact the Labour Relations and Professional Department at headquarters (See Appendix 2).

Revised pay scales do not apply solely to employment within the NHS. Most reputable employers who were previously bound by 'Whitley' should honour the new scales. Practice nurses working in GPs surgeries or working for small scale employers may find themselves subject to tougher negotiation.

An explanatory booklet from the RCN entitled *Understanding Clinical Grading*[6] may be available from your nursing office or the nursing library. Alternatively you can purchase your own copy.

Contracts of employment

When you are offered a contract of employment it is worth studying the fine print and clarifying anything you do not understand. Your entitlement to paid leave and overtime, plus arrangements for being allocated to another place of work to cover for staff absence, should be made clear. If you are unsure or you want to check current staff and service agreements then seek the advice of your trades union via a local steward or

Table 2.1
Advice from the RCN

● Your pay grade on appointment will depend upon the job you will be doing. There is a range of pay scales, nine in all, from A to I. These cover nursing auxiliaries, enrolled nurses, staff nurses, sisters and clinical specialists.

● Credit may be given when determining your commencing salary for completed years of nursing service in an equivalent or higher grade than before the break.

● The clinical grading structure could give rise to some difficulties in deciding whether previous posts held were equivalent or higher than the new grades and it would be advisable to clarify your position at interview.

● Performance related pay, at the moment, applies only to senior managers.

● If you have a problem which is too difficult for you to resolve on your own then as an RCN member you have the choice of going to your local steward, the convenor or any other branch officers, or to full-time officers based at the RCN office for your region.

● The RCN is able to offer you support, advice and protection on professional and employment issues through its network of stewards and fulltime officers. To be able to represent you, however, the RCN has to be 'recognised' by the employer for that purpose and the RCN cannot force any employer to grant that 'recognition'. In places where the RCN is not recognised then representation can only be given as a 'friend'.

● All those whose names are on the Register of nurses maintained by the UKCC are eligible to become a member of the RCN whether they are practising or not.

● The RCN does not issue general guidance to those returning to nursing but is willing to offer advice to individuals if approached.

---

regional office. If you do not belong to a union then ask to see the employer's handbook detailing minimum terms and conditions and ask to amend your contact in advance of signature if you feel this is necessary.

Some employers will include an advisory interview or session with the district finance officer or personnel officer in order to work out income tax and superannuation or pension fund arrangements, or you can request an interview if such an offer is not forthcoming.

When you are working out general costs of working *vis à vis* earning do remember to take into account the costs of studying for any additional qualifications. Your employer may not be able to refund all of your study expenses, particularly if the period of study involved is extensive.

Conditions of work and returning health visitors

When considering an offfer of a job in the community it is worth asking a few questions about the day to day management of the service, and the kind of support you can expect to get from your colleagues.

Reference to the setting up of neighbourhood nursing teams appears in chapter 7, together with an introductory bibliography of suggested reading.

On a practical and down to earth level it is worth finding out what clerical support you are likely to get in the clinic or base where you will be working. Who is there to answer the telephone when you are not there? What assistance and support in managerial and professional terms can you expect from your neighbourhood nursing team manager? What are the aims and objectives of the post? What opportunities are there for group as well as one to one initiatives in health promotion? How is the health visitor's role perceived within the primary health care team, and what approach to their work is taken by medical colleagues working with the neighbourhood nursing team? What specific social problems are prevalent in the area and what support can you expect in trying to prioritise for special need? How much help will you need as a returner in the management of caseloads and identification of priorities within that caseload? What is the continuing education budget post-entry and the employer's commitment to assist you in furthering your own professional commitment?

Professional indemnity insurance for health visitors is available to members of the 17 000 strong TUC-affiliated Health Visitors' Association, the professional organisation and trades union for health visitors and school nurses. More information on continuing education programmes organised by the HVA and other professional advice and activities appears in chapter 4.

There are a limited number of DHA run re-entry courses for community nurses, and some of these may have modules or input designed to assist health visitors back into practice. The difference in costs between HVA two-week courses and DHA courses may be considerable, but not necessarily. It is worth exploring possibilities for both. You may prefer to pay more for a course geared specifically to the needs of health visitors rather than something more general, and may be able to recoup at least part of the costs of attending a course from your local continuing education budget. You may feel that a local course would have more relevance to the job you want or appreciate the opportunity a local course gives you to make new contacts in the district where you will be working.

If there is any possibility of a period of supervised practice before returning to work it is worth taking, in addition to any period of standard reorientation. It will give you the chance to ask questions and get the feel of current practice before committing yourself and will help you to identify learning and professional needs at an early and manageable stage.

Regular meetings with other health visitors for information purposes or purely as support groups can help you to combat the isolation sometimes described by health visitors working in both rural and inner city communities.

Health visitors can be employed in a part-time capacity, and the job theoretically lends itself well to jobsharing. A booklet[7] which includes guidance for managers and would-be jobsharers, as well as a model agreement, can be obtained from the HVA.

Addressing fears and anxieties

Whatever your past experience or clinical area of expertise, you may still feel apprehensive and nervous about returning to practice, even after completing a re-entry programme. It is important for you to have these natural fears recognised and legitimised. You should not be made to feel inferior or unusual because you have respect for your considerable responsibilities.

Coping and support networks can be built up gradually as part of a group exercise and on your own and can provide a forum for discussion and shared experience as well as letting off the inevitable steam and frustration experienced at one time or another. The main inhibitors to progress, and the root causes of fear, can include:

- Unrealistic personal goals and expectations.
- Unimaginative goals.
- Taking criticism of your efforts personally, occasionally being 'super-sensitive'.
- Allowing stress to deplete your resources.
- Fear of failure.
- Lack of appreciation and positive feedback from those around you.
- Fault finding and negative thinking on either side.
- Professional isolation.
- Lack of a peer group.
- Fear of failure or being made to look foolish in front of others (especially patients and junior staff).
- Lack of interest or enthusiasm for the specialty or special problems of patients/clients.
- Trying to take on too much too soon.

Regular support meetings for new staff and course tutors can be arranged informally when a re-entry programme has been completed. This is useful for both parties as problems experienced by returners can be anticipated and dealt with for the benefit of new course members. Meetings need not be addressed by any one person although a specific topic can be aired for discussion if the group wishes. These meetings can provide an opportunity to be sociable and to exchange views and experiences as they arise, and can help to reduce tension and the feeling that you alone have the monopoly on making elementary mistakes.

Keeping up to date with developments in your own specialty can go a long way to adding to your confidence. Attempting to get to grips with all the developments in nursing over the past five years is meat enough for any expert, and you will not be regarded as letting the side down just because you are not familiar with all the latest terminology or research in your clinical specialty.

You will be expected to become more involved in teaching

within your own clinical setting but this does not mean that you have to prepare lectures or notes in advance. Much more is made these days of adding to existing experience and finding solutions to individual problems of patients rather than attempting to apply nursing practice to clinical symptoms and multiple medical diagnosis.

Nursing students are now more accustomed to researching information for themselves than perhaps you were used to, and to asking pertinent questions. What you can expect is to be asked to justify your approach to nursing problems. Very experienced nurses can find this difficult to cope with but are beginning to realise the value of such an exercise in identifying ways of improving care to patients.

Follow up any critical analysis of your work with positive suggestions for improvements. What did you do well and what were your weaknesses? If there is someone at work whose approach to patients or clinical abilities you admire then observe them and use them as a role model. Adapt the best of your practice to the benefit of the experience and see whether you can combine the two successfully.

If you want to you can keep a diary or journal of your progress, rewarding yourself for every new skill mastered or job well done. Make notes on those areas where you feel you need guidance and help, and resolve to seek out that help as soon as possible. Laughing at your own silly mistakes can help to take away any embarrassment and the need to apologise constantly for your gaucheness without any loss of dignity or selfrespect. Patients will often be your greatest ally when testing yourself for the first time.

Sharing your experiences with someone whose judgement you respect and value can help you to place any short term worries in their proper perspective. Membership of a professional organisation and a relevant forum or interest group will help to keep you informed of developments in the field and give you access to study days. It can also help to raise your awareness of new research and any political influences or undercurrents which stand to affect the way services are managed.

Research awareness will keep you one step ahead of changes in policy as related to practice, and help you to field questions from students and other colleagues. Remember that your colleagues need your reassurance too, to confirm that they are doing the right thing. Acknowledge encouragement and assist- ance from them and support them in return. If you find it hard to accept authority from younger nurses who may have less overall experience than you, try to explain your difficulties to them rather than allowing resentment to build up between you. They can feel just as threatened by you and need to have your co-operation as they learn to manage resources and personnel effectively. High handedness may be the result of nervousness on their part which could be defused if you both take the trouble to see the other's point of view. However tempting it may be, try to avoid falling in to the trap of 'in my day we did it this way' or you may receive a stinging reply.

Try to have your progress reviewed regularly with your nurse manager, so that neither of you makes misleading assumptions about your ability to cope or happiness in the job. If you do need to express any dissatisfaction try to do in it a constructive and diplomatic way. She, too, places her professional reputation on the line and any criticism of the clinical environment or her style of management needs to be handled tactfully if it is to receive a good hearing.

Although it may at first feel as though you will always be the new member of staff, or that you will never stop asking questions, most returners express appreciation and gratitude for the support and practical help offered by colleagues, and for the warm welcome extended to them on their return.

Hospital chaplains and your own minister may be able happy to support you through stressful and difficult times, particularly if you are working in an emotionally stressful area. The spiritual resources of patients can do a great deal to help in their recovery or bring about a peaceful death. Acknowledging and respecting the religious observances and convictions of others can help to overcome otherwise distressing or depressing experiences and often succeeds where conventional medical and nursing measures fail. The willingness to share in the experiences of patients; to share their sense of loss, disappointment, anger and grief and the spiritual anguish which can challenge the way they have thought, perhaps believed and behaved in the past, can add to your nursing care much more than withdrawing from or denying such experience. Nurses are no longer expected to sublimate their feelings behind starchy officiousness as has been the case in the not so distant past.

The ability to communicate and to build bridges in human relationships is now recognised as an essential nursing skill; and the opportunity for offering comfort and unconditional acceptance in this way probably has no equal in any other profession.

References

1. P. McEvoy, 'Self-evaluation can protect your competence', *The Professional Nurse*, (1987).
2. UKCC, *The Code of Professional Conduct for the Nurse, Midwife and Health Visitor* (London: UKCC, 1984).
3. R. H. Pyne, *Professional Discipline in Nursing – Theory and Practice* (Oxford: Blackwell Scientific Publications, 1981).
4. T. J. Watson, *Sociology, Work and Industry* (London: Routledge & Kegan Paul, 1980).
5. C. M. Chapman, *Sociology for Nurses*, 2nd edn, Nurses Aid series, (London: Baillière Tindall, 1982).
6. RCN, *Understanding clinical grading* (Harrow: Scutari, 1988).
7. HVA, *Job-sharing: a Labour Relations Guide* (London: HVA, 1988).

CHAPTER 3

Practical Issues at Home and Work

Before taking on any job commitment it is worth looking at your personal priorities in detail, and working out where work will fit in. Although this sounds obvious, it is quite remarkable how many returning nurses remark on the problems of adjustment they encounter once the initial 'honeymoon' period of returning is over.

Having satisfied the urge to 'have a go', they can sometimes be surprised by the everyday practical ramifications of taking on a new job. Nurses who have married or had children since they last nursed may be intellectually aware of what unsocial hours can mean, but if they have not actually experienced them recently they can be caught unprepared. Many of the challenges expressed could be avoided with proper planning and fore-thought. Those I mention here are the most often talked about and may be helpful for some readers.

Working hours

Where possible, seek an employer who is prepared to be flexible. If you have decided to work to a prearranged minimum number of hours, make sure you know which days you will be needed, and whether it is acceptable occasionally to exchange duties with another member of staff. If there are aspects of the job which you would ideally like to share then put these to your manager and discuss possibilties. It is helpful to define these areas in writing so that you both know where you are. Some employers will not allow you to 'job share' officially, but may be open to revising your job description to fit in with local service needs.

If you work less than 37.5 hours every week then you will be classed as a parttime worker. Parttime working does not affect your right to study leave, nor does it mean that you should be given only those jobs which no one else wants. Whatever your commitment in terms of hours worked, you should be able to make a contribution of the same quality as any member of the fulltime staff.

Some employers may encourage you to start with fewer hours than you think you can manage, with the intention of adding to these as you gain more confidence. You may find this frustrating at first, or appreciate the extra breathing space it gives you. It is probably easier to add on extra hours than to take on too much and then find you have to reduce your hours because of outside commitments or for other less foreseeable reasons.

A staff nurse who began by working on an elderly care ward parttime from 9am to 2pm is now working virtually fulltime, despite having five children. Thanks to understanding managers and colleagues the transition has been effectively managed and her service contribution has become invaluable. Her family soon knew what to expect and so the potential for resentment was never allowed to build up.

If your employer has crèche facilities on offer, and your ability to work depends on them, find out well in advance of taking the job what hours the crèche is open, the standard of care offered, and the charges made for the service. Crèches can be expensive to run and it is possible that charges will be prohibitive, particularly if you are returning on a modest pay grade.

You may be limited by the hours the crèche is open as not all remain open in the evening, or begin early enough in the morning. Places may be restricted to certain days, and the crèche may be closed in the school holidays. The competition for places may be fierce where all employees have access to facilities. The crèche may be located some distance away from where you will be working, and some have restrictions as to how far away you are allowed to be from your child in case you need to be contacted. Your child's age will also matter, as there are usually a restricted number of places for babies under one year, depending on the number of qualified nursery nurses available and the design and nature of the building itself.

It has been known for staff to accept offers of jobs on the assumption that crêche places and hours will be organised to fit around the duties of employees. This cannot be taken for granted, however, and it is worth fending off inevitable disappointment by making enquiries before signing any contract of employment.

Transport

If you intend to travel by public transport then do check the reliability of local operators. Since deregulation of bus services some routes may have been altered or replaced. This can matter if you expect to be working late and the bus stage is some distance away from your place of work. You may not want to walk down lonely streets or dark paths alone at the end of a day's work.

It may be possible to share a taxi with colleagues on a regular basis or arrange a lift home. Inter-hospital transport may be able to take you part of the way home, or at least take you to a main thoroughfare away from dark corners.

If you intend to live in a house provided by the local health authority they may be prepared to arrange transport for you. If you intend to live in a staff hostel you may be able to call upon a member of the hospital security staff. Hospitals in inner city areas are sometimes protected by security staff who have an additional responsibility for the safety of residents in staff accommodation.

You may intend to get to work by car or bicycle. If you go by car then you should check on the availability of car parking, as nurses are not generally considered a priority in this respect. Security can also be a problem here, so try to park in highly visible places which are less likely to be jammed by visitors' cars just as you want to get home. Bicycles should have a reliable padlock and carry some form of identification, preferably a police stamp. Your local police station should be able to mark your bike for you.

It is worth estimating potential transport costs in advance and setting these against your anticipated income. If you find you have to put a car on the road purely for your job's sake, by the time you have included petrol, road tax and insurance, plus an allowance for depreciation, that you may be better off working closer to home. Community nurses and health visitors are paid a mileage allowance but you will also want to know who pays for what if you should break down or have an accident, and whether you can claim an allowance against income tax for general depreciation.

Crown cars are used less and less these days, other than in very rural areas. Occasionally you may be asked to share a Crown car with colleagues or even health authority employees from another department. This can lead to occasional problems over who has priority. Check this in advance with your service manager so that you don't risk being caught out when you are in a hurry.

Accommodation

Since the 1983 Rayner Scrutiny of NHS residential accommodation[1] there has been a steady rationalisation of accommodation provided for DHA employees, and this has added to problems for recruiters, especially in areas where private rented accommodation is expensive and in short supply. The sale of land and properties sited in prime development areas has led to a shortage of suitable housing for staff, particularly in the South East of England.

Certain categories of staff have more chance of being offered accommodation, but this may be limited to single applicants living a reasonable distance from the parental home. Preference is generally given to nursing students in their first year of training, and 'younger' staff working in hard to recruit areas. Your employer has no legal or even moral obligation to house you, although they may advise you on what is available locally in the public and private sector.

For advice on buying a DHSS house or flat, on district council and housing association schemes and on special schemes ('hard to let' and low cost home ownership) consult *No Fixed Abode: NHS housing*, a *Guide to your Rights and Options*.[2] This is a campaign booklet which I prepared for the RCN's Association of Nursing Students in 1985; much of it also applies to returning nurses.

Care of dependents

The noun 'dependent' is an ugly label, implying that a person exists only in relation to another person. Unfortunately it now enjoys common usage in social services parlance, and I use it here principally as an umbrella term for those people you may be close to, and have some responsibility for, be they elderly or disabled relatives or friends, children or other family members.

A great many nurses care for dependent parents or grand-parents, and have to juggle their own personal and family needs around long-term commitments. It may be the loss of a partner or the onset of mental illness in a parent which first causes a nurse to give up a successful career in order to care fulltime at home.

When considering the future of a chronically sick, disabled or frail person it is inevitably the nurse in the family to whom everyone turns. Expectations are high, the assumption often being that the vocation experienced by the person who enjoys nursing can be satisfied closer to home. Although for some this may be acceptable as a labour of love, for others it can become an intolerable burden, particularly if the dependent relative or companion is unappreciative or fails to acknowledge the sacrifices being made on their behalf. Guilt or resentment on either side can erode an otherwise loving relationship.

Whether you are married or single, man or woman, the pressure to fulfil your 'obligations' is strong. Different cultures have different attitudes to such obligations; for some it is merely an extension of an already extended family. The British tendency to choose to limit the size of families over the past 20 years, and the need to move around the country in search of better job prospects, has done little to increase the sense of community and neighbourliness which once absorbed so much of the responsibility for mutual support and so-called 'informal' care in the post-war years.

Demands on social services to provide support are rising

steadily as are those made on voluntary groups and organisations who strive to support both carer and cared for with the limited financial and physical resources they have available.

Assistance from the community nursing service, social workers and day or respite facilities can relieve some of the pressure on carers but do not provide any long term solution to the attendant social and emotional deprivation of people living restricted and sometimes insular existences. Years away from clinical nursing can sap the confidence of nurses so that when an opportunity to return to work does come along, individuals feel inhibited from trying to re-establish their careers.

Some enlightened and forward-thinking employers are already beginning to recognise this potential manpower resource for both full and parttime staff.

The experience and resilience of such nurses will be much in demand, not necessarily solely at the qualified nurse level, as the reforms of nursing education begin to be implemented in the early 1990s (see chapter 5). The need to harness and utilise such skills becomes an urgent priority if the NHS is to survive the recruitment and retention crisis so talked about in the late 1980s.

Those responsible for recruiting qualified nurses back into practice should be in the business of welcoming back all staff who have expressed an interest in returning, regardless of age or length of break in service. From my own experience, service breaks of 15–20 years are not at all unusual, although older candidates do tend to underestimate the value of their past experience, apologising for personal inadequacies which, on further examination, do not exist. Such nurses need to benefit from an individual appraisal and assessment of their experience and skills so that re-entry becomes a natural progression for them rather than a hurdle to be jumped.

In evaluations of the length of time spent on supervised clinical allocation before employment, the vast majority of course tutors said that course members felt that time allowed was inadequate, and would happily have continued for longer. Regardless of the amount of time involved it seems likely that staff will always opt for more time if this is offered to them. As one tutor put it: 'The temptation to put off the evil day is irresistible for most people. I have to re-affirm the confidence they are only beginning to find in themselves.'

If you care for a relative or close friend on a longterm basis and feel unable to return to fulltime work it may still be possible to make alternative arrangements in order to work for one or more days or nights a week. Other members of the family may be able to share care by helping out on alternative days or weeks, or over a two day period once a month, so that you can attend a back to nursing course. Some courses run at weekends or in the evenings, and some during school hours.

A popular shift for returning district nurses is the twilight shift – assisting patients into or out of bed – although this may not be what you want for the rest of your life. Residential homes and hostels can accommodate nurses who can only work awkward hours, and who can cover for staff sickness and annual leave. Many voluntary organisations run social and rehabilitation centres which provide stimulating and interesting activities for people confined to home at other times in the week.

If you have a sympathetic employer and GP you could see whether the person you care for would like to come to work with you but spend one or two days a week on a regular basis in a day centre run by the DHA. Social work departments should have details of any local centres and activities, but of course much depends on your relative's wishes and personal preferences. You would probably both benefit in the long term by coming to such a compromise as interests and contacts from outside can save you both from the trapped feeling that a dependent relationship can bring about.

Alternatively you can employ someone to care for your relative at home. Local volunteer schemes may be able to arrange a regular visitor or you could contact an employment agency or advertise for a kindly 'sitter'. The rates of pay which an agency may require vary and are dependent on whether you want someone qualified. Paying another nurse while you nurse yourself may sound dotty, but if both you and your relative can maintain a sense of independence and broaden your outlook on life it may be a worthwhile investment. Placing an advertisement for someone kind and responsible to help may sound an unlikely way to find reliable help but it can have very satisfying results. Early or semi-retired people or housewives looking for a break often welcome a different four walls and a fresh interest.

If you haven't been in touch recently then do contact your GP and health visitor and discuss possibilities with them. If it is not possible to attend a back to nursing course there are various distance learning packages available which can be studied successfully at home. They need not necessarily be any more expensive than enrolling on a course. Even though they are no substitute for practical experience they can at least familiarise you with current terminology and introduce you to contemporary nursing philosophies.

Community mental handicap and mental health teams are now much more geared to supporting carers as well as clients, and would be glad to offer any help they can. If you have struggled alone for some time you may be pleasantly surprised at what is now available to you. Contact your local community health council by letter or telephone and ask to be put in touch with whoever is responsible for your area. This may be easier in the long run than trying to hack your way through the jungle of your local community health or social services departments. CHCs are very consumer oriented and can provide an enormous range of explanatory leaflets and basic information.

Alternatives in child care

If you have exhausted the possibility of an employer's crêche facility then you may want to consider the alternatives, which are usually childminding or employing a nanny or au pair. Reciprocal arrangements with another nurse or friend can work – so long as you are flexible and no money exchanges hands, but if you have a child under five and payment is involved then your 'childminder' will either have to register with the local authority (that is if she cares for your child in the minder's own home) or be employed as a nanny in yours.

If you can find someone like yourself who is in the same position then this can be an ideal arrangement. Not only do you go to work knowing that your child is in safe hands, but you have a ready made friend, sympathetic listener and companion for you and your child all in one neat package. The potential saving compared to paying for a childminder can be considerable; more so for a nanny.

Shared nannies are becoming more popular and other children can provide stimulation and company if yours is an only child. Local branches of the National Childbirth Trust are a good source of information on nanny shares. The costs of employing even a shared nanny, however, should be thoroughly investigated beforehand. Rates in London and the South East may be prohibitive as qualified nannies (NNEBs) are much in demand but in short supply. Women in better paid jobs can negotiate better conditions especially for nannies who live in.

Au pairs' hours have to be fitted around language classes and travelling and so are unlikely to fit in with yours, unless you are prepared to compromise a great deal and have the energy after work to deal with the appalling homesickness experienced by young people living far from home.

Finding a suitable registered childminder is probably the only option available to most of you as even the best nursery schools and crêches can seldom offer the kind of hours you are likely to need throughout school holiday periods. If you have children of school age you may be able to depend on a neighbour, relative or friend to do the necessary fetching and carrying and occasional early suppers. Substitute 'grannies' sometimes advertise their services in local newspapers or shop windows, and can be reliable. If you do rely on a friend or neighbour on a fairly relaxed and informal basis it is worth showing them some appreciation occasionally, a return of favours or a thoughtful gift. Being taken for granted is the biggest cause of disillusionment with this kind of relationship and a sincere gesture every now and again can help to keep it sweet.

Lists of registered childminders can be obtained from the under-fives adviser employed by the social services department. Under the Child Minders Regulations Act of 1948 a person caring for reward for one or more children under five years of age to whom they are not related is required to be registered with the local authority.

The childminder will be investigated for any previous criminal convictions and have her home inspected for cleanliness, adequate space and 'reasonable safety'. Such inspections are theoretically repeated every two or three years, although I have come across some childminders who have not received a follow up visit for several years.

It is up to parents to satisfy themselves as to the suitability of a childminder, and the social services department are not likely to want to become involved over minor issues. They will want to know about a childminder who fails to provide a safe environment or where children appear to be neglected or ill cared for. The arbiter of taste in this instance has to be parents themselves, and much can be done to avoid unhappy experiences from the outset by determining preferences and approaches to the care of your child when your childminding arrangement begins.

The actual payment at time of writing is between £1.50 and £1.70 per hour per child, but with a possible reduction for any second and subsequent child. This may include meals but not of the kind or quality you may prefer. You can choose to take packed lunches for your child if you want to. The best childminders are usually well known in the area and come recommended by friends or colleagues. Those who are new to childminding can take a while to become established, however, so do not assume several vacancies to be a reflection on the childminder herself. Professional jealousy between childminders is quite common, and so it is worth getting an independent opinion if you find one minder putting down another without evidence of a good cause.

It is worth discussing your child's needs in detail and having a few rehearsal sessions before committing yourself to a job. Do not do as I did and arrange to work only to find that the childminder changes her mind within the first few days.

Ask to see your childminder's certificate of registration and find out how many other children she will be caring for in addition to yours. Does she employ extra help if necessary? How much space and what kind of play equipment does she have? What is her attitude towards tantrums or bad behaviour and what action would she take on your behalf? Make your requirements on such things as physical punishment, sweet eating and so on clear from the outset.

Is she approachable and easy to talk to, or do you find yourself apologising to her for forgetting things or because your child has heaps of energy? Does your child have an unusual and relevant medical history, such as convulsion or allergies, and would she know what to do in an emergency? Inconsistencies can be very confusing for young children and conflicting attitudes over toilet training and discipline can lead to frustration and unhappiness.

Always leave details of where you can be contacted – even if you only intend to be away from your usual number for a few hours – and provide your child's full name, date and place of birth, and your GPs name, address and telephone number. An organised childminder may well ask you to complete a form giving such relevant details, and should at least ask you for them.

When you are satisfied that your child is happy and cared for then don't hesitate to make the most of a good childminder. The rate of pay is such that she must be genuinely fond of children to want to put up with them day after day!

Single parents may find that they have priority over places in state run nurseries. If you are in this position and you want to return to work it is worth making enquiries of your health visitor or the local authority under-fives adviser.

References

1. DHSS, *NHS Scrutiny Programme: Residential Accommodation in the NHS* (London: DHSS, 1983).
2. A. Morton-Cooper, *No Fixed Abode – NHS housing – A Guide to your Rights and Actions* (London: RCN, 1985).

Recommended reading

Caring at Home, a handbook for carers (London: Kings Fund).
Taking a Break, a guide for people caring at home. (Newcastle Upon Tyne: Taking a Break).

CHAPTER 4

The Back to Nursing Movement and Prospective Employers

The back to nursing movement has established itself over the past five years, partly in response to a national shortage of qualified staff, and partly as a result of the UKCC's stated commitment[1] to introduce mandatory updating programmes for nurses and health visitors returning to practice after a specified minimum break in service. Initiatives on recruitment and retention of staff were highlighted by a major national campaign run jointly by the Department of Health and *Nursing Times* in 1988.

Director of nursing policy and practice at the RCN, Derek Dean, addressed hard-pressed managers in his book *Manpower Solutions*[2] published by the RCN in 1987. In his advice on 'bringing back the lost', he targeted two groups for re-employment; those who had originally left nursing because they were 'uninterested for one reason or another', and those who had left to have children.

He pointed to demographic changes in the population, a lack of competitiveness among health authorities as a labour market, and a labour turnover in which the profession renews itself numerically every six years as part of the explanation for the shortfall in establishment figures.

The declining number of nurses in training leading to a reduced output of qualified staff, fewer 18-year-olds as a pool for recruitment, and a massive retention problem in London all contributed to a need for concerted action, he stressed. In calling for an 'unprecedented management' initiative to offset the effects of reduced staffing levels, Derek Dean did not mince words: 'It is not an over statement to say that a crisis is imminent and can only be averted if action is taken by all concerned as a matter of extreme urgency.'

The evidence to date is that DHAs and independent sector employers are taking Derek Dean's predictions seriously, and are preparing to defuse the demographic time bomb by revamping their image to attract the attention of potential returners, and by setting up re-entry schemes which will help to instil confidence in staff who feel nervous about coping with new and demanding roles.

Nursing agencies have often been the means to re-entry in the past, and they too are having to adapt to new forces at work which for them could represent a consumer boom.

Preparing for your return

The chances are that you belong to one of the groups Derek Dean has identified. Your motivation and skills have already been considered in the previous chapters. What you need to know about now is how to bring your practice and your registration status up to date, and the different routes of re-entry available to you.

The law and re-entry programmes

As this book goes to press (April 1989) there is no law which requires nurses or health visitors formally to update their practice before re-entry. Significant moves have been made towards introducing such a requirement in the near future, however, and it would be prudent to take account of these when planning your return.

UKCC guidelines of good practice

Charged with the setting up of a central UK single professional register of nurses, midwives and health visitors, and mindful of its responsibilities for enhancing professional standards, the UKCC first began looking at the issue of mandatory refreshment for nurses and health visitors while still a shadow body in 1982.

Following the report of its working group, recommendations concerning this were passed on to the newly appointed UKCC on its inception in July 1983. Having considered this report the Council went on to state its commitment to the provision of approved re-entry programmes in its first annual report of December 1984.

A period of consultation with the professions followed, and in May 1986 the UKCC published an important document entitled *Guidelines For Good Practice – Return to Practise Programmes for Nurses and Health Visitors.*

Those employers who were already geared to providing some form of re-entry course for returning nurses then had the benefit of these guidelines to work from, and began adapting their course objectives and outcomes to the recommended UKCC criteria. The document clearly helped employers to identify what they hoped to achieve by running such programmes, and sowed the seeds which will eventually culminate in a nationally recognised curriculum in the future.

A further consultation paper issued by the UKCC in September 1988[3] took proposals a stage further. Responses to a questionnaire sent to NHS authorities in March 1988 had shown that only 8 per cent of employers requires nurses and health visitors to undertake re-entry programmes before employment, even though individuals might have had substantial breaks in service.

Eager to build on the positive response to the earlier guidelines, and to impress on employers their collective responsibilities in assisting returners to practise safely, the UKCC put forward the following proposals for consideration:

● 'following a break in practice from a post requiring a nursing or health visiting qualification of three (since modified to five) years or more, a re-entry programme will be required in order for a person to return to practice'.
● The minimum length of such a re-entry programme should be set at 144 hours throughout the UK.
● On completion of a suitable programme outcomes based on up to date knowledge of practice of nursing or health visiting must be achieved by a returning nurse or health visitor.

(These outcomes had already appeared in draft outline in the earlier *Guidelines*, but were now modified and revised following the response to consultation.)

- Courses offered should be provided by employing authorities on a full or part-time basis, and could include appropriate distance learning material.
- To ensure that a minimum UK standard is met, the National Boards should undertake the approval of programmes.
- Provision for re-entry programmes should be linked with periodic relicensing to ensure safe practice.

Certain changes in the rules contained in the Nurses', Midwives' and Health Visitor's Act (1979) are needed to make updating a legal requirement, and these must be put before Parliament as with any law reform. Given the remaining time left open for consultations within the professions and the time needed to enact rule changes, the requirement is unlikely to reach the statute books before 1990.

The other thorny issue to be addressed is that of course funding. At present many courses are funded by DHAs, while the cost of others is met by returners themselves. Much depends on the length of courses and how comprehensive they are. The cost of evening courses or those consisting of a few sessions in a school of nursing cost considerably less than residential week long courses or part-time variations held over a period of several months.

The wide range of courses in terms of content and timespan presumably reflects the budget and teaching staff available and the demand created by service needs (notably shortage of staff in specific areas), and the needs expressed by interested applicants.

As employers respond to the guidelines set out by the UKCC then parity of courses will emerge and budgets for courses will need to be arrived at in response to local situations.

If employers are to be expected to meet the cost then they (and the Department of Health) will have to be convinced that moneys invested in providing programmes will have a worthwhile outcome in terms of better recruitment and retention of staff.

The UKCC has the moral high ground: it can argue that such

courses must be funded in order to ensure safe practice and to protect the vulnerable public from nurses or health visitors whose practice is out of date and potentially dangerous. Certainly various options in providing funds will have to be looked at, and some agreement reached if mandatory refreshment is to become a reality.

In practice many returners already pay some contribution towards courses. In my early research for this book it was evident that where applicants paid a fee to attend a course, the attendance and completion figures were significantly higher than where courses had been provided free of charge. Some assistance has been provided by local sponsorship and training grants (formerly from the Manpower Services Commission) have been made available. The independent sector has also contributed to developments in the area by setting up courses aimed at recruiting staff back to work.

Estimates of the number of returning nurses are difficult to gauge accurately on an annual yearly basis, although the UKCC has placed an educated guess through manpower enquiries at 2500 a year.[4]

Whether or not you will be asked to pay for your course remains at the discretion of course organisers and managers, therefore, and I am unable to give any hard and fast guidance here, other than to say that they will have to be kept at a reasonable level to be affordable, particularly by those who have been unemployed or bringing up a family.

Although at the moment it is up to you to decide what form of updating you would like to undertake, it would be useful to look at any developments in your area aimed at your special interest, and to find out from employers what they might expect from you in advance of offering you a job. Advice on how to go about this appears later in this chapter. I would first like to explain your obligations on an issue which has caused a great deal of concern and confusion for returners by being made to appear much more complicated than it actually is.

Periodic fees and re-licensing

In July 1983 the UKCC single professional register absorbed the registers and rolls formerly administered by the General Nursing Councils. Records in England and Wales and Northern Ireland, however, still held the names and addresses of many who had long ceased to practise, some of them no longer alive, and so the records as they stood could not be described as 'live'.

In a massive postal exercise the UKCC updated these records. You may have received a letter from them early in 1984 asking for up to date details. From January 1987 a system of periodic licensing was introduced, whereby nurses, midwives and health visitors wishing to remain on the SPR, and so maintain their eligibility to practise, must pay a periodic fee every three years. This keeps the register 'live' and provides a steady income for the UKCC, so helping it to move towards financial independence from government subsidy.

So even though you may have paid what you thought was a once and for all registration fee on qualifying prior to 1983, if you wish to remain eligible to practise you are now required to update your registration status with the Council if you have not already done so.

At the time of writing the fee stands at £30 for a three year period. If for some reason the UKCC has not caught up with you then you can write to the Registration Department, United Kingdom Central Council for Nursing, Midwifery and Health Visiting, 23 Portland Place, London W1N 3AF, and you will be sent standard forms to complete.

Depending on your employment situation and the length of time you have had away from nursing you may be asked to provide a character or employer's reference. On payment of the requisite fee your qualifications will be validated and your up to date details recorded on the SPR.

Once your registration status is up to date you will be sent a plastic card containing your name and Personal Identification Number (PIN) and it is this card which constitutes evidence of your 'licence to practise'. When you apply for a job, your prospective employer will ask you to produce this card so that he may be satisfied of your eligibility to practise.

One of the advantages of such a card over paper qualifications and former GNC registration badges is the protection it offers against the possibility of fraudulent use.

Scotland has enjoyed a system of periodic relicensing prior to the appointment of the new statutory bodies in 1983, and so those of you previously registered with the GNC for Scotland will already be familiar with the practice of periodic relicensing, and will be quite accustomed to what has become the subject of some controversy south of the border.

New titles for nurses, midwives and health visitors

Table 4.1 illustrates the new titles for those entered on the constituent parts of the UKCCs Single Professional Register. These were introduced in July 1983 when the new statutory bodies for the professions came into being. Practitioners may use former titles as a matter of courtesy, although this is becoming less usual.

All those entered on parts 1, 3, 5, 8 and 9 of the SPR are now described as first level practitioners, while those entered on parts 2, 4, 6 and 7 are described as second level practitioners. The professional competencies required of first and second level nurses are commensurate with the level and duration of initial nurse training, and these are examined more closely in Chapter 7 when discussing changes in nursing practice generally.

Registered health visitors must have a first level qualification in order to undertake postbasic health visitor training. Those entered as registered midwives may be first level trained nurses who have gone on to take additional postbasic training as a midwife, or may be direct entrants to midwifery, in which case their qualification is at first level.

Linking re-entry to relicensing

By the early 1990s it is envisaged that nurses and health visitors wishing to relicense will have to provide evidence of either current employment requiring a nursing qualification or the successful completion of a re-entry programme approved by the National Board of their country of practice.

In this way the UKCC not only keeps a 'live' register of practising professionals, but ensures that they are not placed in the vulnerable position of attempting to give care without sufficient up to date theoretical and practical knowledge. Standards of care should therefore be safeguarded and protected and the possibility of nurses being inadequately prepared for their roles should reduce dramatically.

Table 4.1
The Single Professional Register (SPR)

Parts	New Title	Former Title
1	Registered General Nurse (RGN)	State Registered Nurse (SRN)
2	Enrolled Nurse (General) (EN(G))	State Enrolled Nurse (SEN)
3	Registered Mental Nurse (RMN)	Unchanged
4	Enrolled Nurse (Mental) (EN(M))	State Enrolled Nurse (Mental) (SEN(M))
5	Registered Nurse for the Mentally Handicapped (RNMH)	RN for Mentally Subnormal/ Deficient (RNMS/D)
6	Enrolled Nurse (Mental Handicap) (EN(MH))	State Enrolled Nurse for Mentally Subnormal/Deficient (SEN(MS))
7	Enrolled Nurse (EN)	Those trained as enrolled nurses in Scotland and Northern Ireland
8	Registered Sick Children's Nurse (RSCN)	Unchanged
9	Registered Fever Nurse (RFN) Training for this specialism is now obsolete and so this part of the register is now closed to new admissions	Registered Fever Nurse (RFN)
10	Registered Midwife (RM)	State Certified Midwife (SCM)
11	Registered Health Visitor (RHV)	Health Visitor (HV)

Approval of current re-entry programmes

The curricula and finer details of National Board approved programmes still have to be fully considered and agreed. This does mean that re-entry or back to nursing courses presently operating will not necessarily be approved retrospectively for the purpose by the National Boards. Any course you choose to undertake before updating is made mandatory may not later satisfy the Boards if you decide to delay return to nursing or health visiting in the meantime.

The likelihood is that if a current course meets the UKCC's criteria then the National Board may consider an exemption from the new rules, although this again will have to be allowed for in legislation. The problem is that the Boards would have great difficulty in assessing the standard of a course retrospectively, particularly if it has had no dealings with it previously.

If you do not intend to return to nursing employment in the near future, then you can only remain as up to date with nursing theory as possible in anticipation of your planned return, and hope that the evidence you eventually provide of recent study is sufficient to convince the Board of your readiness to return.

It would still do you no harm to attend a re-entry programme in the meantime, as it will give you a taste of current nursing practice, and help you in deciding exactly what you would like to do in the future.

Course supervision

The best action open to you at the moment is to undertake a re-entry course which conforms to the criteria outlined in the UKCC's *Guidelines for Good Practice*. The National Boards will probably oversee and approve their own courses once a formula for these has been finalised for standard and content by the UKCC. However, each National Board will wish to evolve re-entry programmes with their own country's needs and priorities in mind, and this may be reflected in the modus operandi of individual boards, and the considerable amount of time and discussion which will no doubt take place in advance of reaching a UK wide agreement.

Scotland, for instance, already has a flourishing and well-established system of continuing education and personal development for those already practising. the demographic differences for instance in recruitment and retention problems reflects the number and nature of re-entry programmes held in different parts of the UK. The present trend of setting up courses only in response to staff shortages will be superseded in the future by any forthcoming legal requirement, and so the administration of courses and the rationale behind them will have to change accordingly.

The existence of a firm strategy for continuing education may, in theory, preclude the need for re-entry programmes as they exist at present, and it is the job of the members of each National Board to align continuing education needs with the UKCC's own policies regarding the maintenance and improvement of professional standards as laid down in current legislation. Whatever is ultimately decided by the boards and the UKCC it is still in your own and your patients interests for you to undertake some form of formal updating, even if for the moment this is left to your own and your employer's discretion.

Before going on to look at re-entry and back to nursing courses in detail I would like to consider alternative routes of re-entry available to you first.

Alternative routes of re-entry

There are several routes open to qualified nurses and health visitors, although these will be limited if you wish to remain within one area of clinical practice.

These include returning:

● Via a back to nursing or re-entry programme organised by your local health board or district health authority. This is unlikely to guarantee you a post on completion, but most employers will be happy to discuss possible openings or vacancies with you, subject to satisfactory references and your suitability as assessed at personal interview.
● Via a back to nursing course organised by a nursing employment agency. Employment opportunities will be discussed at some time during or before the course. Some agencies may waive the fee if you register with them on completion of a course.
● Via full or parttime work in a private nursing or rest home, or as a resident or non-resident nurse in an independent school or college.
● Via a post working privately in the patient's own home.
● Via a residential post in a community house, hostel or institution.
● Via work arranged for you by a nursing agency.

- Via registering for work with a nurse 'bank' in the NHS or in the independent sector.
- Via full or parttime employment in the NHS, but without completing a re-entry course prior to take up such employment.
- Via work in charitable organisations and institutions.
- Via private clinics.
- Via working as a practice nurse in a GP surgery or group practice.
- Via employers abroad.
- Via teaching or research in tertiary and higher education establishments.
- Via retraining for a new specialty requiring your original qualification for entry.
- Via work in occupational health nursing in industry or commercial organisations.
- Via employment in the independent health sector, which includes hospices and charitable trusts as well as large hospitals and hospital corporations.

This list is not intended to be exhaustive, and certainly does not include areas where your nursing qualification is used indirectly, such as working as a children's nanny or as a sales representative for a pharmaceutical or product manufacturer.

Before making a decision about your preferred route of re-entry it is useful to study the desired outcomes for nurses and health visitors completing a re-entry programme suggested by the UKCC. Given the length of your own break in service, and any efforts you have made to update yourself in any or all of these areas, would you feel confident to return to practice tomorrow?

Most of you will probably want to qualify your answers. If you have been out of nursing or health visiting for six months or less you may feel that completing a formal course is a waste of valuable time which might be more profitably spent in reorientation to your new job.

If you have accepted a job offer it is still worth enquiring whether there are any local 'refresher' courses operating as part of in-service and continuing education. You may be able to arrange day or shorter release periods for any study days or short courses relevant to your practice which would also help to bring you up to date.

Do not take a job on the basis of a vague letter of appointment. Examine and agree on a job description first and a contract of employment which you are satisfied with and understand. For advice regarding clinical grading see chapter 2. Remember to take out professional indemnity insurance against any possible action for negligence or malpractice and see whether there are any professional organisations or societies which serve your clinical area. Continuing education tutors and nursing librarians are a good source of information on special interest groups and forums, as are the journals. Appendices at the end of this book will provide you with some contact names and addresses.

If you do not feel ready yet to return to practice without attending a re-entry programme there is no need to feel inferior or cowardly compared with friends who are more confident. What follows is general advice applicable to either group on finding information about job and training opportunities, and on responding to local recruitment drives.

Return to practice and re-entry programmes

Where to find help and information

At the time of writing there is no central source or register of information regarding re-entry programmes. Advice on continuing education is available from several organisations and these may have to be approached individually in order to put together a picture of opportunities available to you locally. The situation on provision and supervision of re-entry courses is unique to each member country of the UK, and so what follows is advice relevant to your country of intended practice. There is no reason at present why you cannot take a course in one country even though you intend to take up a job elsewhere. The approach to such provision is not yet uniform, however, and so entry requirements and any formal assessment of your competence at the end of the course may differ according to local recommendations and practices.

Scotland

For information on re-entry courses in Scotland write to: **the Nursing Recruitment Adviser, Scottish Health Service Centre, Crewe Road South, Edinburgh EH4 2LF** (telephone 031–332 2335). Advice on courses provided by individual health boards and colleges of nursing can be obtained from this address, but if you have a particular query concerning local provision you can either contact your local college of nursing direct, or write to the chief nursing officer at your local health board for clarification.

The Health Service Centre should be your first port of call for all general career enquiries as it disseminates information on both basic and postbasic nursing education. The careers centre has a library which is open to nurses and other health service staff. Opening hours are Monday to Friday from 9am to 5pm at the address given above.

Wales

For information on re-entry courses available in Wales you are advised to contact **your local district health authority**. If you have difficulty in obtaining the information you want then write to: The Chief Nursing Officer, Welsh Office, Cathays Park, Cardiff CF1 3NQ, or to the Nurse Adviser, Post-basic Education, Welsh National Board for Nursing, Midwifery and Health Visiting, Floor 13, Pearl Assurance House, Greyfriars Road, Cardiff CF1 3AG.

England

For advice on courses available in England write to: **Mrs Jean Heath, English National Board Careers Service, PO Box 356, Sheffield S8 0SJ.** A process of rationalisation and joint initiatives with establishments of higher education makes identifying local schools and centres of nurse education quite difficult unless you are familiar with local mergers and health authority politics. If you are familiar with your local school of nursing then you can write directly either to the director of nurse education or to the tutor for postbasic education based at the school.

Northern Ireland

If you would like to undertake a course in Northern Ireland you are advised to contact the director of nurse education at your **local college of nursing,** or write to the chief administrative nursing officer at your **local health board** for details of local initiatives.

Miss E. N. I. Lamb,
CANO,
Eastern Health and Social
Services Board,
12–22 Linenhall Street,
Belfast BT2 8BE.

Miss P. Donald,
CANO,
Western Health and Social
Services Board,
15 Gransha Park,
Clooney Road,
Londonderry BT47 1TG.

* Mr W. Black,
CANO,
Northern Health and Social
Services Board,
County Hall,
182 Galgorm Road,
Ballymena, BT42 1QB.

Mr F. Rice,
CANO,
Southern Health and Social
Services Board,
20 Seagoe Industrial Estate,
Craigavon BT63 5QD.

Non NHS courses

Details of courses for returners organised by nursing agencies or commercial conference organisations appear in the national weekly nursing press from time to time and in local newspapers. Courses may also be advertised in local jobcentres and public libraries or on the display boards of local employment agencies. Some agencies may also circulate details to nurses currently registered with them.

Appropriate terminology

The formal title given to back to nursing courses is 'return to practice programme' or 're-entry programme' as advised by the UKCC. The actual title of the course matters a lot less than the content, but a word of caution is necessary here to help you differentiate between programmes designed to prepare you for re-entry to the profession, and those which may be open to nurses currently practising, namely 'refresher courses'.

Refresher courses are generally aimed at updating nurses in particular specialties or all nurses on one particular topic, such as wound care, nursing research or pharmacology. Such courses may be of interest to you as a returner but they are not the same as re-entry programmes, and would not be recognised for the same purpose if you ever had to provide evidence of an updating course to your National Board.

Mandatory refreshment (as in re-entry programmes) for re-turning nurses and health visitors is a separate but related issue to refreshment of practitioners already in the service. Employers are sometimes guilty of blurring or confusing the two. Some hope to provide one kind of course with the intention of killing the two proverbial birds with one stone. The learning needs of the two groups are quite distinct from each other, however, and you should take care to establish exactly what is on offer before accepting a place. Refresher courses are usually one or two day affairs as opposed to a formally planned and evaluated re-entry course, and should not be used as a cheaper alternative to providing a structured re-entry programme.

Tailoring a course to meet your needs

Most employers will be only too happy to help you tailor your preparation for re-entry to your own learning needs and those of the job you hope to take up. When applying for a place on a re-entry course keep the following questions in mind so that you can compare what is on offer to your own best advantage.

● What are the specific aims of the course?
● Who is responsible for planning the course and how is it assessed?
● Do the hours fit in with your existing commitments?
● What fee is charged and must you finance this in whole or in part?
● Is it possible to have the fee reimbursed if you consequently

take up employment/register with the employer organising the course?
- Is there an organised syllabus? If so, what does it cover?
- Does the course take due regard of the UKCC's *Guidelines for Good Practice?*
- What support is available to you from tutors and other staff?
- What is the clinical content of the course? Is clinical practice supervised and formally assessed before course completion?
- Will you have an opportunity to meet nurses who have already completed a similar course whether they have returned to practice or not?
- What preparatory reading (if any) is expected of you prior to attending the course?
- How much private study is assumed in addition to attending the course?
- Does the course lead to a certificate of completion or competence and if so, what value would such a certificate have on the job market?
- Will job opportunities and interview skills be discussed at some time during the course?
- Will you be offered a contract of employment while attending the course, and what is your position regarding professional indemnity insurance while undertaking clinical practice allocations?

Course content

The content of courses varies widely, and is usually arrived at by the demands of the service. The course should be general in nature if it is to comply with UKCC criteria, but it may have an additional specialist component aimed at preparing nurses for work in different clinical settings.

Courses for health visitors provided by the HVA are geared much more to the needs of that group, and these are discussed on pages 67–9.

At present re-entry programmes range from three evenings to six months' day release plus supervised practice, and so it is virtually impossible to list every variation on the theme here. The difficulty for anyone returning after a break is gauging just how up to date the teaching methods and philosophies of care are in any one school of nursing. It has been shown that some schools offer a rehash or revision programme based on pre-registration modules, while others prepare courses in line with the very latest developments available. If you have not kept up with the nursing journals or have been out of practice for a long time then you will have to trust to luck or the recommendations of others as to the relevance and value of any course you choose to attend.

If returners are to be able to comply with the desired outcomes as defined by the UKCC's guidelines then the course offered would have to satisfy requirements set out in Table 4.2.

If you study the UKCC's Code of Professional Conduct (Appendix 1) you will see that the criteria for desired outcomes relates directly to what is expected of the registered nurse and health visitor. They are also very closely related to the competencies required of registered nurse in the Nurses' Rules (Nurses, Midwives and Health Visitors Act, 1979). These are reproduced in chapter 7. Taken together, all these requirements constitute a set of minimum professional standards by which individual practitioners can be assessed and judged.

It seems logical that the minimum required of any returning nurse or health visitor should be that of any other registered practitioner. By satisfying the requirements of the UKCC *Guidelines*, therefore, your skills will be easily as good as any newly qualified nurse, and given any previous nursing experience you may have had, probably much better. The implications for raising standards of care in the profession are tremendous if employing authorities can succeed in meeting the desired outcomes of the UKCC in centres throughout the UK.

If the course described to you seems to bear no relation to these criteria do make further enquiries. It may be that a new course is still in the planning stages, or that what you want is offered at another local centre. Some employers are only just getting round to formalising recruitment and retention policies – and all that goes with them – it may be that you are one step ahead of them in attempting to update yourself appropriately. It does no harm to let them know of your interest while a course is in preparation.

Some employers may not run courses for groups of returners

Table 4.2

According to the latest available information from the UKCC, *it is proposed that on completion of a suitable programme, the following outcomes, which are based on up to date knowledge of the practice of nursing or health visiting, should be achieved by the nurse or health visitor in order to practise safely after a break in service:*

Desired outcomes

1 The ability to initiate and carry out emergency procedures effectively and as appropriate.
2 The ability to measure accurately, record and understand the relevance of patient/client data obtained by personal observation or through the use of equipment.
3 The ability to administer medicines safely.
4 An understanding of factors within the environment which relate to the safety of patients/clients, their families/friends and colleagues.
5 The ability to design, execute and evaluate plans of patient/client care, based on appropriate models.
6 An understanding of the practitioner's educational role in relation to patients/clients, relations/friends and colleagues.
7 An understanding of the current issues and educational programmes which affect professional practice.
8 The ability to use appropriate communication skills in relation to patients/clients, relatives, and other members of the care team.
9 An understanding of appropriate current legislation, guidelines, codes of practice and policies.
10 An understanding of the current structure of health and social services, resulting lines of authority and responsibility.

In order to meet these requirements it is expected that the programme will include both theoretical and practical components.

---

but instead offer to help you plan a personal programme of study aimed at satisfying the same requirements. These can be just as useful even if you do not have the benefit of an instant peer group with whom to celebrate or commiserate on your shared experience.

If you do intend to follow your own programme see whether you can find a 'mentor' or other suitable person to whom you can go for encouragement and guidance when you need to, rather than attempting to battle it out on your own. You can also ask to be put in contact with others in a similar position to yourself and if you want to you can always arrange to meet regularly or form a support group to discuss matters which are relevant to all of you in your day to day work.

Course contracts

Temporary contracts of employment may be offered to you if you attend a course which has a high clinical input. Courses operating in this way tend to be held on a system of day release or modules which include actual shifts in wards or departments.

Employers may offer such contracts with a view to making them permanent once they are satisfied that you have completed the course successfully. Take care to establish whether within the terms of such a contract you are considered part of the rostered qualified workforce, or whether you are to be treated as supernumerary.

The implementation of the 1988 Clinical Grading Review as outlined in chapter 2 is complex, and you will need to clarify your position as regards your entry point on the scale. The grading should reflect the actual responsibilities of the job, and any additional qualifications and experience you bring to the job: follow the advice given on contracts and job descriptions generally and be careful to establish what the parameters of the contract are before you agree to it.

Re-entry programmes for health visitors

Courses aimed at community nurses and health visitors have been relatively late arrivals on the 'back to nursing' scene. A few are designed to take in aspects of all community specialties, including district nursing, community psychiatric nursing, community mental handicap nursing and health visiting. They are run by DHAs and in general cost much less than those run by the Health Visitors' Association.

The latter's courses are, however, particularly geared to health visitors and school nurses, are residential and more intensive than courses offered by DHAs. They are also apt to be more authoritative, having been planned and organised by a professional organisation which also has a very important role in labour relations. The HVA has an on-going annual programme of continuing education courses available to health visitors and school nurses open to members and non-members. It has also pioneered a two week residential course for returning health visitors which takes place on two separate weeks with time allowed for preparation and consolidation of practice in the interval between component parts (Table 4.3).

Details of planned courses and current fees are available from: **Education Officer, Health Visitor's Association, 50 Southwark Street, London SE1 1UN (telephone 01–378 7255).** The HVA's annual study conference usually takes place in the autumn and this can provide members with a focus for current health visiting issues. All HVA members receive a free monthly copy of the journal *The Health Visitor*. There is an excellent library at HVA headquarters which can be utilised by post, and which does not close its doors to non-members as some other libraries do.

A substantial preparatory reading list of recent reports and other material of relevance to health visitors is available from the education officer at the HVA. Subscriptions to the quarterly HVA 'current awareness bulletin' may also be arranged by contacting her at the address given above.

Details of membership and annual subscriptions for health visitors and school nurses may be obtained by writing to the membership secretary at HVA headquarters.

Information and advice on health visiting as a career can be obtained from recruitment officers at the addresses given in Appendix 3.

If you are a member of the RCN you can also write to the RCN Adviser in Primary Health Care at RCN Headquarters, 20 Cavendish Square, London W1M 0AB. Specialist forums served by the Association include: Community Nurse Managers Forum; District Nurses Forum; Family Planning Nurses Forum; Fieldwork Teachers/Practical Fieldwork Teachers Forum; Health Visitors Forum; Liaison Nurses Forum; Practice Nurses Forum; School Nurses Forum. Special interest groups include chest clinic nurses, coronary heart disease specialist nurses and tuberculosis visitors.

Table 4.3
Example of content of residential course for returning health visitors

Part 1
Day 1
  Developments in the health services.
  Practices and principles of health visiting.
  Neighbourhood nursing.

Day 2
  Aspects of nutrition.
  Child health surveillance.

Day 3
  DHSS benefits.
  Free afternoon and evening.

Day 4
  Systematic health visiting.
  Law and the health visitor.

Day 5
  The immune system – immunology in practice.
  Plenary session and evaluation.

Part 2
Day 1
  Nutrition and diet.
  Weaning.
  Behaviour problems in schoolchildren.
  A report back on a systematic approach to health visiting.

Day 2
  Report writing and centile charts.
  How to get out of the 'Yes, but . . .' syndrome.
  Minor ailments.

Day 3
  Child abuse and neglect.
  Free afternoon.

Day 4
  Child sexual abuse.
  Senior citizens and empowerment.
  Approaches to healthy ageing.
  Health visiting and middle age.

Day 5
  Caring for the carers.
  Evaluation of the course and plenary session.

Re-entry via a new nursing specialty

It is always possible to return to nursing by studying for a specialist qualification. It is sometimes necessary to have previous experience in the clinical area before secondment on a clinical nursing studies course can be arranged, or for previous experience to have some direct relevance for future work. For example, if you have ambitions to work as a district nurse it may help to have worked in the care of elderly or disabled people. Voluntary work in the community can be just as useful as anything you may have done in a paid capacity.

Information on postbasic training leading to another first level qualification (RNMH, RMN, RSCN, RGN) is best obtained from nursing careers advisers (addresses appear in Appendix 3). Help in finding your way around postbasic opportunities via clinical nursing studies courses and other aspects of career development can be found in Jill Baker's book *What Next?*

If you are familiar with your local school or college of nursing then you can write to the director of nurse education for information on courses run, entry requirements and availability of places.

Finding the right job

Job fairs and forums

National job fairs or forums are held in different parts of the country to attract nurses into jobs of every possible variety. Employers in both public and private sectors can hire exhibition 'stands' with display boards advertising job opportunities on offer. Talks and meetings on topics of interest to nurses looking for a change in career direction are held throughout the day, and personnel and recruitment officers make themselves available to answer questions and arrange interviews for interested applicants.

Such fairs are a great morale booster for any nurse who feels unappreciated. Suddenly there are hundreds of people just waiting to improve her career prospects! Some career conventions have crèche facilities arranged. Recruitment videos are sometimes shown, and advisory sessions may include applying for jobs, interview techniques, and general issues related to job hunting.

Job fairs are usually very lively and informal, and you can roam at leisure, surveying what is on offer and gathering literature on jobs you might not have considered in the everyday run of things. Admission is usually free. Advance details are published in the nursing press (see Figure 1) and local radio advertising is often used at the time of the event.

Local recruitment drives

These are usually much more modest affairs. They may be advertised in local newspapers or on local radio. Interested nurses may be invited to an informal gathering over coffee, or to a structured recruitment day addressed by speakers and rounding off with an open session devoted to local job vacancies.

Members of staff are often available for an informal chat, and this can be a golden opportunity to absorb the general atmosphere and the attitudes of prospective colleagues.

Such recruitment drives can be organised by NHS managers or employers in the private sector. The latter can usually be distinguished by the more generous hospitality – cheese and wine parties are very often the province of a nursing recruitment agency, or other private sector employer. It is worth investigating all the opportunities on offer before coming to a decision. The managers of nursing agencies have often had considerable experience in assisting nurses back into practice after a career break, and can be extremely helpful and conscientious in responding to any doubts and queries you may have.

The approachability of NHS authorities will largely be determined by their current recruitment situation. In Scotland and Northern Ireland, for instance, the shortage of qualified staff simply does not exist on the same grand scale as in some parts of England, and central London particularly. For this reason managers may be less experienced in dealing with returning nurses and health visitors.

If you intend to move to a new area to take up employment it is wise to do some homework on local factors affecting recruitment. It may be that the cost of living and paying rent locally is

CAREER CONVENTION PROGRAMME
22–24 NOVEMBER 1988, OLYMPIA, LONDON

TUESDAY 22 NOVEMBER

Chair: Patricia Collinson.
Nursing Officer Department of Health

POSTBASIC OPPORTUNITIES

10.15	Midwifery
10.30	District nursing
10.45	Health visiting
11.00	Education
11.15	Mental illness
11.30	Mental handicap
11.45	Paediatrics
12.00	Special hospitals

CONTINUING EDUCATION

12.15	Department of Health video
12.45	Open learning
1.00	ENB courses
1.15	Discussion
1.45	Close

WEDNESDAY 23 NOVEMBER

Chair: Patricia Collinson.
Nursing Officer Department of Health

POSTBASIC OPPORTUNITIES

10.15	Midwifery
10.30	District nursing
10.45	Health visiting
11.00	Education
11.15	Paediatrics
11.30	Special hospitals
11.45	First steps to management
12.00	The independent sector
12.15	Agency nursing
12.30	Nursing overseas

CONTINUING EDUCATION

12.45	Open learning
1.00	ENB courses
1.15	Discussion
1.45	Close

CAREER DEVELOPMENT

5.15	Department of Health video
5.35	Three talks on nursing careers with questions
	Education
	Research
	Management
7.15	Close

THURSDAY 24 NOVEMBER

Chair: Meriel White.
Nurse Recruitment Officer, City and Hackney Health Authority

NEW HORIZONS

10.15	The independent sector
10.30	Agency nursing
10.45	Long term care
11.00	First steps to management
11.15	Research
11.30	Nursing in the Army
11.45	Nursing overseas

MAKING THE BEST OF YOURSELF

12.00	How to apply for a job you want
12.20	How to present yourself at interviews
12.40	Your questions answered
1.00	Close

See you there!

Figure 1
Sample career convention programmes (Reproduced by kind permission of *Nursing Times*, from issue 9 November 1988)

prohibitive, or that the hospital is due for closure in the forsee-
able future. The standard of NHS accommodation available to
trained staff is variable, and even if you are happy to put up
with this in the short term, in the longer term it may have
adverse effects on your personal life or hopes of a future career.
I have met some very disillusioned nurses who responded to
vigorous recruitment drives and travelled many miles from
home, only to find that they were expected to live in dilapi-
dated, out of the way nurses' hostels with no hope of raising the
funds for anything better in the vicinity. Redundancy, too, can
be a threat, particularly where large psychiatric or mental
handicap hospitals are being sold off as property which is excess
to requirement.

Be aware of these issues when attending an interview or open
day, and never accept a post without seeing for yourself what is
actually being offered. Some employers recruit on the basis of
interviews held in hotels as visiting recruitment forums. Most of
them are very reputable, but do be cautious about promises
which sound too good to be true.

Jobcentres

Department of Employment Jobcentres have branches in most
towns and cities and some may display nursing vacancies. It
appears to be at the discretion of each branch to decide how
nursing vacancies are publicised. I rang ten different Jobcentres
on the same day, and received ten different responses!

Most will usually be able to provide you with a contact name
and address, but if this is no help, then you can contact the
personnel officer at the district health authority's address.

Classified advertisements

Most private sector employers use the classified section of local
and regional newspapers, and the national nursing press.
District health authorities may also produce their own regular
bulletins prior to using the classifieds.

If you want a general survey of the job scene, *Nursing Times*
leads the field. Its classifieds cover NHS and non NHS appointments, plus jobs in higher education, research and industry.

Nursing agencies and overseas recruiters also advertise. *Nursing Standard* produces handy supplements, which have recently included material on back to nursing, agency nursing, nursing in the independent sector, nursing abroad and working in London. Your local nursing library may hold reference copies of these.

Prepare to be confused by the plethora of different job titles: unremitting reorganisation of the NHS and changes to the statutory framework for the nursing and midwifery professions have wrought havoc. There is a book to be written on the identity crisis apparent in nurses who have been left to the mercy of all the changes, and you will be far from alone if you cannot tell a facilitator from a patient services coordinator!

Nurse banks

Nurse banks originated in hospitals which required a pool of available trained staff from which to draw in times of staff shortage.

Not all DHAs operate a bank, but those which do usually welcome applications from returners, and are happy to discuss your mutual requirements at an early stage. You will be asked to state your preferred days and hours of work, and whether you are willing to be called upon at very short notice to cover for staff absence or other emergency.

Some nurses are very enthusiastic about the bank as a route of re-entry, as it enables you to sample different wards and departments and introduces you to new people. You very soon become familiar with the layout of the hospital and its policies, and can perhaps identify one area where you might like to work permanently.

You may be asked to cover for staff sickness, or study leave, or find yourself particularly busy during peak holiday periods. You must be prepared for all eventualities, however, and not find yourself being asked to take charge in an area where you have insufficient clinical knowledge and experience. When you first apply to join the bank, make clear to your employer just how much responsibility you feel able to take, and discuss ways of improving your clinical and management skills to take on additional responsibilities.

If you agree to work in an area which is unfamiliar to you, discuss the role you will be expected to take with your nurse manager. It may be that with adequate supervision and a period of reorientation it will not take very long to prepare yourself for a new role, but do take care to acknowledge your limitations, and to make known to your manager how these are likely to affect the care you give.

If you have another parttime job, or domestic commitments, then bank nursing can be a very flexible way of keeping up to date professionally. Be sure to fill in time sheets correctly and to let your manager know as soon as possible if you are unable to work as arranged, or be available on call. Even if you only work for a few hours a week, take out professional indemnity insurance. COHSE, the RCN, and the HVA all offer indemnity insurance schemes, and your local steward should be able to provide you with specific written details of this. (Health visitors should contact their local HVA centre, or the labour relations department at headquarters.)

Agency nursing

The old-fashioned, rather genteel, image of nursing employment agencies has been superseded by much more streamlined, commercially aware organisations run with a mixture of personnel expertise and crisis management. They are often fiercely competitive, and have a vested interest in establishing a reputation for reliability to both employees and employers.

Many towns and cities have high street branches of the bigger agencies, while smaller operations may operate from more modest premises and be run individually or in partnership. Agencies advertise locally in newspapers, and may carry regular advertisements in the national nursing press. The term recruitment consultants does imply 'high flyer' and this description may lead you to organisations with an interest in placing nurses in particular specialties, in management positions, or abroad.

The Nursing Agencies Forum at the RCN is evidence of the agencies' rise to respectability, and it is no longer the case that 'those who can, do; those who can't, work for agencies'. It is the agency's job to establish a good working relationship between employers and agency staff, and it is in your interests to promote this by fulfilling your obligations to both by working in a professional and reliable way.

When you first approach an agency check that they are registered as an employment agency with the local government authority. Every reputable agency should display a certificate of registration for the benefit of the public and those who register with them.

Membership of the Federation of Recruitment and Employment Services Limited is a good sign, as FRES has a code of practice which ensures the right level and number of qualified recruitment staff to assist and advise you. The code protects against misleading or unethical advertising and provides a surety that you are given full, written details of what registration with a particular agency involves.

Terms and conditions of employment, including rates of pay, should be discussed at the outset, together with your qualifications, past nursing experience and level of expertise, and availability for work. Some agencies like you to wear their own distinctive uniforms. Will you be provided with free uniforms, or do you have to purchase these for yourself?

Enquire about your income tax position, as this will be influenced by what you earn with the agency plus any other parttime or freelance work. If you elect to become self-employed you will have to let your local inland revenue office know. Agency staff may be able to advise you about certain tax allowances, such as travelling expenses, uniform, indemnity insurance, subscriptions to the journals, and to a professional organisation.

Your main concern may be getting work in a post commensurate with your past experience and abilities. Most agencies will discuss this with you before accepting a job on your behalf, and will be sympathetic to your needs. Any agency which places you in an unviable or potentially dangerous position could be accused of negligence by delegation, and so it is equally not in their interests to place you inappropriately. If you work regularly for one agency you may want to have your position and experience reviewed from time to time, so that future work you undertake can be constructive and part of bona fide career development. Some enlightened agencies run back to nursing and refresher courses. They will usually have to charge for these, but you may be reimbursed if you subsequently register with the agency or fulfil a certain number of hours working for the agency.

Occasionally agencies work under contract to one hospital or authority, and you may find yourself becoming a semi-permanent fixture in one post. You may prefer the flexibility over hours this offers, but you should weigh the pros and cons regarding working for an NHS employer and sickness pay, holiday pay, pension, study leave and so on. If you are offered a fulltime post by an employer who has been introduced to you via a nursing agency, you should consider the etiquette and ethics involved of leaving the agency to go to work for one of their clients, thus depriving them of their commission from employers. Read the small print of any agreement you have with an agency, and be honest with agency staff about your dilemma. It is not unusual to be in this position, and it may be that there is an accepted procedure to follow in the eventuality of employers making you an offer.

Tony O'Malley, an experienced agency nurse, has the following general advice for anyone contemplating working for an agency:

'There are several problems a nurse returner might face when working for an agency, and it may be helpful to be aware of these in advance. Nurses working for agencies may often be telephoned and asked to undertake an assignment that they do not feel very confident about. The caller from the agency may plead and cajole you into agreeing to accept the job, especially if it is a last minute booking and they are desperate for someone.

'Nurses should be advised to resist such pressure and not be afraid to turn down any assignment which they feel may be outside their sphere of competence. Don't give in to comments such as "You are very choosy", or are "always turning down work", or even "Do you really want to work?". Remember that you are self employed and a free agent.

'It is the agency's responsibility to find you the type of work you have indicated that you are interested in. If you only want certain types of work and your agency is not able to supply enough work to suit you, then feel free to register with other agencies at the same time. Many agency nurses do this and it poses no problems.

'When you do accept an assignment from one agency, be sure to inform the other agencies that you will not be available for however long the accepted work takes. This will be much appreciated because it saves agency staff time and effort in trying to find you work unnecessarily.

'It is also possible that an assignment you accept turns out to be different from what you had been led to believe. This may be because the client has misinformed the agency, or has redefined your duties prior to your arrival. I am aware of agency nurses who have turned up at a hospital expecting to work on a ward caring for elderly people, only to be sent to work in the intensive care unit. It is also not uncommon for hospitals to request a number of nurses from an agency without detailing the areas the nurses will be required to work in until they report for duty. It is wise to be alert to this, and to stand your ground if asked to work in an area which is beyond your present capabilities.'

Independent sector employment

When discussing the independent health sector, many nurses describe a one dimensional perception of what is involved, namely a private hospital, luxuriously furnished, with demanding clients and a price list to match. The reality is in fact much much broader than this, and as you can see from the following list, there are a wealth of opportunities providing care and comfort for all sectors of the population.

● Hospices.
● Private clinics, ranging from gynaecological and fertility clinics to general practice, alcohol or drug dependency, dermatology, sports injury clinics.
● Occupational health posts in industry, or large commercial companies, retail outlets and corporations.
● Residential homes, including nursing and rest homes, community houses and hostels, children's homes.
● Independent schools and colleges.
● Private hospitals offering acute or longterm care.
● Charity and consumer advice agencies.
● Private home nursing.
● Teaching and lecturing on a freelance basis.

- Running employment agencies.
- Large multi-national corporations in the USA and the Middle East.
- Hospitals run by charitable trusts.
- Staff training and development for private sector employers.

No list can be exhaustive, but it can give you an idea of the range of opportunities open to you. Most private sector employers advertise locally and in the nursing press, although some may run recruitment drives of their own, or exhibit at a job fair.

The individual employer's attitude to returning nurses will probably be the major deciding factor for you, even if pay and conditions are high on the list. Much will depend on the ability of the employer to offer you optimum conditions for job satisfaction. If the staff : client ratio is low and the environment for care well equipped and attractive, then you will have to measure this against the breadth of experience which represents your alternative within the NHS. Study the non NHS sections of *Nursing Times* and *Nursing Standard* and this will give you the most up to date information on current vacancies.

Job applications and interviews

The procedure for job applications and interviews is well known to most returners and I have therefore assumed that you do not need detailed guidance on this. Initial applications for jobs need not include a separate employment history (curriculum vitae) unless this is specifically requested in a job advertisement. Most employers will only ask you to repeat this information in a standard application form anyway.

A tidy, polite letter of application expressing your interest, date and level of qualifications, and details of your most recent employment is all that is required in the first instance, together with evidence of your registration status.

If the job or employer is unusual, then it may be helpful to go into more detail in advance of your interview, simply to allow whoever is vetting your application to pick you out from the crowd. As an employer myself I have often found the best employees to be the most straightforward on paper. Those who promise great things do not always match up to their own or anyone else's expectations!

References

1. UKCC, *Annual Report* (London: UKCC, 1984).
2. D. Dean, *Manpower Solutions* (London: RCN, 1987).
3. UKCC, *Consultation Paper: Proposals for Statutory Requirement for Nurses and Health Visitors to Undertake Re-entry Programmes prior to their Return to Practise* (London: UKCC, 1988).
4. UKCC, *Counting the Cost*, Project Paper 8 (London: UKCC, 1987).

Recommended reading

'Agency nursing', *Nursing Standard* Special Supplement, 16 July 1988.

J. Baker, *What Next: Postbasic Opportunities in Nursing* (Basingstoke: Macmillan Education, 1988).

J. Booth, 'Applying for a job or course', *The Professional Nurse*, **3** (1988) pp. 473–4.

J. Englefield, 'Part-time staff: a blessing in disguise?', *The Professional Nurse*, **3** (1988) pp. 524–6.

'Independent health sector nursing', *Nursing Standard* Special Supplement, 27 August 1988.

'Nursing Abroad', *Nursing Standard* Special Supplement, 17 September 1988.

J. Rogers, 'Clinical career structures – a lot to consider', *The Professional Nurse*, **3** (1988) p. 377.

CHAPTER 5

The NHS and its Mid-life Crisis

The cause of British nurses and nursing itself in the 1980s has been championed most consistently by Trevor Clay. As general secretary of nursing's largest trade union and professional organisation, the Royal College of Nursing, he has succeeded more than any single politician or political agitator in raising the public's awareness of the critical role of nurses in maintaining the nation's health.

He has calmly continued to assert the nursing voice, adroitly altering the popular subservient image of the nurse to one of deep political and personal conscientiousness as the patients' advocate and closest ally.

Steering the RCN through the gravest provocation and confrontations – over industrial action, inadequacy of resources, management reorganisations, and the latest débâcle over the implementation of a new clinical grading structure – he is strategically well placed to voice a considered opinion on the future of the profession in Britain as we enter the next decade.

In his book *Nurses, Power and Politics*,[1] he charted the progress of the nursing cause, looking at issues of conscience, education, image and professionalism as the NHS prepared to celebrate its 40th anniversary.

Clay has no doubt that the nurse's professional life is compatible with being political:

> Participation in the political life of the country is the alternative for individual nurses to the silent frustration of the past or industrial action. . . . Each day we spend working with people we see their needs and the services they deserve.

He urges nurses to look beyond the immediate frustration of not being able to give all that they would wish for today's patients, but to resolve as individuals to do 'everything reasonable within our power and through our nursing organisations to make sure that tomorrow's people get the nurses and the nursing they deserve. I am confident that together we can be a powerhouse for change.'

Trevor Clay retires in 1989, sadly on the grounds of ill health, and his determination and incisive leadership is a very great loss to the profession. His 'powerhouse for change' is both optimistic and courageous, coming at a time of unprecedented change and innovation in the NHS.

Rapidly advancing technologies in health care and clinical practice taking place across the whole spectrum of medical, surgical and mental health specialties depend for their success to a large degree on the sufficiency of sound nursing skills and personnel.

Increasing and conflicting demands made on funds for NHS use tends to focus media interest on the service's shortcomings rather than its strengths. Headlines describing the 'mid life crisis' of the NHS have done little to promote its image as a positive and worthwhile employer.

As Dr David Owen says in his book *Our NHS*,[2] by exploiting and accentuating the apparent weaknesses in the system, the media is at risk of endangering the survival of the whole service by making it unattractive to recruits of the right calibre and commitment:

> Those who cynically exploit the current problems of the NHS and yet who purport to support its purpose ought to pause and reflect upon the effect of some of their activities in creating a mood of pessimism about its future. The deficiencies of the NHS need to be dealt with away from the headlines . . .

It is certainly true that the climate for attracting new recruits to the professions is not improved by continued reporting on the doom and gloom aspects of working in the NHS. The rolling stone effect of perpetuating negative thinking, rather than positive constructive action, is to lower morale at a very critical and potentially exciting stage in the development of nursing.

Nursing into the 1990s

There is no doubt that by returning to nursing in the next decade you will be helping to prepare the profession for the enormous demographic and social challenges facing Britain in the 21st century. The proposed reform of nurse education in the UK, which received approval in principle from the Conservative government in May 1983,[3] promises a period of tremendous upheaval as the delicate balance of educational and service priorities is carefully weighed and restructured. But with upheaval comes renewal, and an unrivalled opportunity to grasp the nettle nursing's leaders have talked about for years: an opportunity to redefine and reshape the parameters of nursing itself.

Visions of the nurse practitioner of the future are ambitious and exciting. In an effort to prepare nursing for meeting society's needs in the future, policy makers have challenged many of the traditional views and approaches of nurses who evolved in a very different social milieu, and instead identified a much broader role for the new practitioner aimed at improving standards of care available to the public. The hope seems to be that nurses will be better prepared and better enthused to address the nursing needs of society without the shackles placed on them by an outmoded system of training.

Before going on to discuss the reforms known as Project 2000, it might be valuable to describe the recently introduced statutory framework for nursing, midwifery and health visiting as a background to the report.

The current statutory framework for nursing, midwifery and health visiting

When the Nurses, Midwives and Health Visitors Act 1979 came into force in July 1983, nine statutory bodies which had previously governed the professions were replaced by the United Kingdom Central Council for Nursing, Midwifery and Health Visiting – and four National Boards, one for each constituent country, England, Northern Ireland, Scotland and Wales.

The UKCC is charged with responsibilities for establishing

and improving standards of training and professional conduct. It also maintains the Professional Register.

Registered nurses, midwives and health visitors of the four countries elect members to the National Boards every five years. Additional members are appointed to the National Boards by the Secretary of State. 1979 Act requires the Board to identify seven of its members to serve on the UKCC. The Secretary of State appoints directly 17 members to the UKCC. Officers of the council and representatives from the Health Departments also attend council.

National Board members meet regularly to discuss and agree on matters relating to the provision of education and training and the implementation of policies at local level. It is the job of the Boards to approve and advise institutions which provide programmes leading to registration as a nurse, midwife or health visitor, and to implement the UKCC's policy requirements.

There is a degree of autonomy within each of the four countries, and although they may unite in the same objectives (such as improvements in educational and professional standards), each has to be responsive to the nature and demands of its country of origin. Within the parameters of kind, standard and content of programmes studied by the UKCC the influence of elected practising members of the professions is beginning to be felt.

The UKCC and National Boards have a very important function in regulating standards of conduct by practitioners. Those alleged to be guilty of misconduct such as to question their continued right to practise may become the subject of consideration by the Investigation Committee of a National Board and, where necessary, be referred for a hearing before the UKCC's Professional Conduct Committee (PCC) to answer the charge of being unfit to practise.

The PCC has the power to remove practitioners found guilty of misconduct from the Register, and to restore them within the terms of the empowering Act. Those who are alleged to be unfit to practise by virtue of illness can be referred by the Investigating Committee, Professional Conduct Committee or any concerned citizen to a separate UKCC Health Committee, so that their cases may be considered with medical reports and advice available.

Any citizen (whether within the profession or not), may allege misconduct or unfitness due to illness. Those who are removed from the Register by the Professional Conduct Committee or Health Committee and are aggrieved by that decision may appeal to the appropriate Appeal Court for the part of the UK in which they reside.

Project 2000 – a new preparation for practice

The UKCC's radical review of education and training, entitled *Project 2000 – a new preparation for practice*,[4] usually known as Project 2000, was presented to Council in the Spring of 1986, and a period of consultation with the professions followed.

A detailed analysis of the 2000 responses to the document was later published, as well as a financial consultancy analysis of manpower, finance and implementation issues. In the main, the UKCC's proposals had two principal elements: a package of education and training reforms, and a package aimed at improving manpower supply and retention.

Members of the original project team took as their starting point the anticipated health care needs of the society in the 1990s. Heralding Project 2000 as a landmark in nursing history, UKCC chair, Audrey Emerton, described the proposed reforms as designed to produce more appropriately prepared nurses equipped to meet the perceived health care needs of future generations,[5] Despite the inevitable uncertainties and anxieties which such major change might represent, she stressed the need for investment in education and training, and for more effective manpower planning and deployment if health care in the UK was to be put on a stronger and more confident foundation:

> 'Many nurses, midwives and health visitors would like even more radical changes, but the UKCC's (present) strategy will:
>
> ● Provide the necessary levels and types of nursing care and which Government plans and Health Authorities' strategies demand.
> ● Reflect the principal aspirations of the professions to provide better care.
> ● In the medium term prove to be more cost-effective.

- Maintain the pre-eminent position of British nursing in the world.
- Address issues of finance and manpower realistically.'

The debate over Project 2000's cost and manpower implications has raged ever since the project group reported, but there is a strong consensus of feeling that the time for radical change is now at hand. The recommendations of Project 2000 should be read in full in order to appreciate the rationale behind them. Copies are obtainable by post or to personal callers, from UKCC offices at 23 Portland Place, London W1N 3AF.

Space available here permits only a summary of the main points of Project 2000. Any re-entry or reorientation programme will usually include a discussion based on the UKCC's video presentation of its final proposals. Courses of preparation for the new Project 2000 type education and training are in the planning stage. The implications of these reforms for all nurses, midwives and health visitors are enormous. A period of adjustment will be required as the role of support workers is properly identified and established. Until the UKCC's final recommendations have definite government approval, accounts and impressions will remain the subject of speculation.

Summary of recommendations

1 A new division of labour characterised by a new single level of nurse who will embrace much of the work of the present two levels of nurse.
2 The introduction of a new specialist practitioner to undertake specialist roles in the hospital and community setting. (Such specialists will have a greater degree of experience, and have completed additional education and training; their qualifications may be disease linked, ie diabetic liaison, stoma care, or may represent specialist knowledge in nursing intervention or in health promotion. Some specialist practitioners will combine teaching with their practice and some will be team leaders.)
3 A new list of competencies for the new nurse will be enshrined in statutory rules.
4 A new programme of preparation for the new nurse will normally be completed within three years, and will begin

with a Common Foundation Programme (CFP) of at least 18 months in length, followed by a branch programme in mental health; or nursing of persons with mental handicap; or nursing of the adult; or nursing of the child.

5 The UKCC proposes to maintain the present 18 month post-registration education and training for midwives and to maintain separate and distinct competencies for midwives. It will continue to give support and encouragement to the extension and development of 3 year direct entry programmes.

6 The introduction of supernumerary status for nursing students. In future students will be under the control of the Education rather than the Service side, and will only make a service contribution of 20 per cent of the student's time (approximately 6 months of the 3 year period).

7 The introduction of non-means tested NHS controlled grants for nursing students, with provision for higher grants to be made available to mature entrants.

8 The cessation of the enrolled or second level nurse training as a move towards a new single grade of nurse.

9 Wherever possible nurse teachers will be required to be graduates. The overall aim is to improve the education and training environment so that a teacher/student ratio of 1:12 will be realised, and that 'the facilities available for education and training should be no less than the best provided in higher education establishment'.

10 The introduction of a new range of nurse helpers/support workers in the clinical setting to assist the qualified workforce in their duties.

Many first level nurses (although still a minority) now undertake basic nurse education as part of undergraduate study for a degree in nursing, social or life sciences. Joint initiatives at all levels of pre- and postregistration courses are now being introduced, and more qualified staff are choosing to study for a qualification at diploma or degree level as part of their continuing professional education. It is envisaged that the role of the clinical teacher as such will be subsumed into a wider role of teacher practitioner, who may have additional specialist knowledge and who is likely to be ward or unit based.

The single most contentious issue contained in Project 2000 is the cessation of preparation of new enrolled nurses. The status of the second level nurse has troubled the profession for years, not least because they have been depended on as the mainstay of practical bedside nursing, while being expected to take on more responsibility than their training prepared them for. As part of the move towards a single grade of nurse, enrolled nurses who wish and are able, are to be encouraged to convert to first level nurse status by way of a conversion course or some other approved means of study and assessment of competence.

The UKCC expressed its concern in a paper published in September 1988,[7] stating that it was 'extremely concerned and aware of the difficulties experienced by large numbers of enrolled nurses in securing a place on existing conversion or bridging courses'.

Of course, not every enrolled nurse will want to, or be academically capable of, converting to first level status. The UKCC accepts this, and has indicated that all those who wish to remain as second level nurses should not be disadvantaged in the pursuit of their careers.

Recommendations on the additional preparation for conversion are included in the UKCC Paper PS & D/88/05, *The Enrolled Nurse and Preparation for Re-entry to a First Level part of the UKCC's Register*.[7] Your local director of nurse education will hold a copy, and your local nursing library should have one on file. Alternatively, copies may be available by writing direct to the director for professional standards and development at the UKCC.

In principle, courses may be specially designed for ENs on a full or parttime basis, or 'comprise an individually designed range of approved learning activities, which might include day release, distance learning components, contract learning and planned modules from existing first level nurse courses'.

Conversion courses must address the kind, standard and content of courses required by the UKCC prior to application for registration as a first level nurse. These are discussed in chapter 7.

When applying for entry to a conversion course, past experience and qualifications will be taken into account, of course, but the demand for places on the 52-week courses is such that returning nurses are likely to be disadvantaged from those already practising.

The UKCC insists that any second level nurse seeking entry to a first level part of the register must successfully complete an examination of the same standard as that required for students undertaking a three year first level nursing preparation. All conversion courses must be approved by the National Board of the country of practice.

Recognising the sheer impossibility of providing an adequate number of conversion courses of the 52 week full-time mode, the UKCC has outlined a more flexible approach to the problem by allowing for appropriate course content arrived at in ways outlined by PS & D/88/05. Whether the commitment from present enrolled nurses exists to make such approaches feasible, and whether there is sufficient financial help available to put them into practice, remains to be seen.

If, as a returner, you prefer to remain as a second level nurse, there should be no problem in obtaining a place on a re-entry programme. Some fears have been expressed over the possibility of employers discriminating against ENs in favour of first level nurses. Conversely, it is thought that some employers will leap at the chance of employing enrolled nurses knowing or believing them to be a cheaper alternative in terms of pay. The clinical grading structure is such that enrolled nurses should never now be considered as a cheaper alternative. The grading applies to responsibilities inherent in the post, so a job requiring the management skills of a first level nurse will not be open to those with a second level qualification.

The structure and grading is now very sensitive and complex, and any advice I give here has to be responsible and realistic. I do not want to mislead you, or to deter you from making the right personal decision.

The appointment of ENs over first level nurses is a matter for local interpretation by nurse managers, for which there are really no obvious hard and fast rules. Make clear to your prospective employer any plans you have for the future, and make sure that the post you accept is appropriate to these. If you are a member of a union you can seek the advice of a steward. RCN members are also advised to write to the college's assistant adviser (enrolled nursing), Susan Scott, at 20 Cavendish Square, London W1M 0AB, for advice and an information pack on issues of interest to enrolled nurses.

Nursing in context – who sets the standards?

At present the most accessible personal means we have of assessing the standard of care we give to patients is the UKCC's Code of Professional Conduct.[8] The current legislation states that: 'The powers of Council shall include that of giving, in such manner as it thinks fit, advice to nurses, midwives and health visitors on standards of professional conduct.'[9]

In November 1984 the UKCC addressed the professions directly when it published and circulated the second edition of the Code. Reg Pyne, director for professional conduct at the UKCC, has suggested six definitions of the Code[10]:

1 That for registered nurses, midwives and health visitors the Code is an extended definition of professional accountability.
2 That it is one means by which the UKCC seeks to satisfy the requirements of the law.
3 That the Code is a portrait of the kind of practitioner the Council wishes to see within the professions.
4 That the Code is a backcloth against which allegations of misconduct and unfitness to practise are judged.
5 That it is a weapon with which practitioners can fight for improvements in standards, and the elimination of risks in the interests of their patients.
6 That the Code is a statement to the profession of the primacy of the patients' interests.

The Code appears in Appendix 1. It is worth re-reading it before continuing with this chapter.

When you begin to read about contemporary nursing practice you will soon become familiar with the issues surrounding the 'exercise of professional accountability'. But what exactly is it, and what relevance has it in every day terms?

Burnard and Chapman[11] warn that the words 'accountability' and 'responsibility', although often used synonymously, are actually quite different:

> While people may be held to be responsible for an action they may not always be asked to *account* for it. The nurse, however, is not only responsible for the care given, but should be able to explain why it is given in the way it is. It is necessary for the nurse not only to be concerned with the outcome of the action but she must understand its origins and the process of carrying it out.

Learners, for instance, may not be held accountable, because accountability implies knowledge, and it is unlikely that the learner will have acquired sufficient knowledge or have sufficient practical experience on which to base the assessment of the care given.

The student may therefore be held responsible, but not accountable, for her actions, until she becomes sufficiently knowledgeable and experienced, and hence qualified.

Burnard and Chapman go further than this definition, by recommending that knowledge should be research based and up to date if it is to be the best for accountability in practice.

In their book *Professional and Ethical Issues in Nursing* they carefully consider each clause of the Code of Conduct, and expand on its scope and implications. The authors see the requirement for the nurse to re-register every three years (periodic licensing), as an important step forward in ensuring 'that all patients receive the highest level of care and that the qualified nurse can really be seen to be in a position of accountability'.

If we define accountability as 'being answerable' to someone for our actions, then to whom are we answerable? Even 10 years ago any nurse who was asked this question would probably have replied 'I'm answerable to sister.' Today the reality is just as straightforward, but may not be what a returning nurse might expect.

The UKCC's global accountability is to the public on behalf of the professions. The nurse's individual accountability is to her patients first, but additionally to her managers, her employers and to her profession. Thus, where a conflict of interest exists between satisfying the wishes of the manager/employer and protecting the interests of the patient, your duty of care is to your patients first.

This has raised far reaching and important issues of conscience since the Code was first published. Nurses are now encouraged to exercise their professional judgement in safeguarding the interests of individual patients and clients, and for some this means exposing poor management and refusing to carry out instructions which they believe to be against the interests of their patients/clients.

It can take a great deal of courage and confidence to challenge colleagues in this way, but as you will see by studying the Code itself, the definition and standards of conduct required are clear and unequivocal, even if putting them into practice is not always as easy as it is made to sound.

Those of you who trained under a very autocratic system, dominated by a strictly imposed hierarchy where nurses came somewhere close to the bottom of the pyramid, are likely to find the concept of accountability quite daunting. Whatever your length of time away from the bedside, however, the Code of Conduct enables us to make sense of accountability, and to assess its relevance to the settings in which we work.

As Reg Pyne advises[12]: 'In summary the portrait (Code) is of a practitioner who has the capacity to challenge, the honesty to ask why, the empathy to care, the skill to perform competently, and the determination not to be put down'.

Copies of the Code, plus guidance on confidentiality, and on advertising by registered nurses, midwives and health visitors, are available as advisory pamphlets from the UKCC.

Tutors and mentors will wish to examine and introduce professional and ethical issues relating to the Code as and when opportunities present themselves. The references and further reading I have included here would make useful introductory reading to this subject and may help to prepare you for sessions and discussions based on the concept of accountability.

The nature of stress in nursing

A graphic account of the cumulative effects of too much stress experienced by nurses is given by Martin Bamber[13]:

A nurse under stress cannot listen empathetically nor respond sensitively. Stress in the nurse can erode the nurse–patient relationship, or even act as a barrier to forming one. The quality of care provided by the nurse can be influenced by the levels of stress among the work force.

While most of us would acknowledge that some level of stress is required to enable us to function and to be sufficiently motivated, the effects of continued high levels of stress have been shown to have a damaging effect on the ability to maintain our personal sense of purpose, usefulness and well-being.

Bamber blames glamorised media portrayals of nurses for contributing to the problem in that they 'do nothing to support realistic expectations of working in a hospital, but only seem to strengthen the "angel" stereotype'.

As Bamber explains, such high expectations of the work, and an unrealistic idealism surrounding 'caring' and the medical model of illness, 'come crashing down with the reality of work experience'.

Stress is a subject which has received a lot of attention and study in recent years. If we consider sources of stress as 'stressors' which build up to form a number of pressures, then it becomes possible to identify where stress is coming from and what it can ultimately lead us to. We can then begin to look for stress reducing and coping strategies to help alleviate the difficulties experienced in the everyday work situation.

Potential stressors

Looking at stress generally, and not necessarily as it affects nurses, the following might be considered as potential trouble spots:

● Transition and change, particularly major personal life changes and catastrophes, such as bereavement, separation, divorce, financial hardship, illness, the birth of a child (to include miscarriage and stillbirth) conflict in relationships at home or work, having 'something to hide', working to deadlines, taking up a new job, moving house, taking examinations.
● Threats to our sense of dignity and self-worth, and to our authority or control over a situation.

93

- Burdens of responsibility, worry over those close to us, our children, elderly parents, the health or welfare of a spouse.
- Performance stress – do we meet other's requirements as a husband/wife/mother/daughter/son/employee? Who assesses our performance, and how much store do we set by their judgement?

Thinking more specifically about nurses we could include:

- Conflicts of interest in trying to serve two masters (the patient and 'the system') and shortcomings in preparation and instruction for a new role.
- Conflict between 'managing' and being managed.
- Pressure to 'cope', and not be seen to let the side down. Pressure to live up to our own and other's expectations.
- The need to deal with tragic, emotionally traumatic and depressing situations, and to help others to acknowledge and come to terms with loss.
- Increased workloads, lack of recognition for the standard of work achieved, lack of feedback and appreciation, being taken for granted.

The inadequacy of nurse training in the past to equip nurses for these pressures and the consequences of pressurised decision-making is a very good reason in itself for reforming nurse education. As Jane Salvage points out,[14] nurse training to date has done very little to make nurses into strong and independent people:

> Everyone in nursing has at some time experienced the abuse of power by someone more senior, and has been hurt by it, yet the system is difficult to modify.

Strength and independence are useful prerequisites in defending ourselves against the effects of stress, but they need the support of a communal sense of responsibility, of sharing a load, and of sharing it fairly in order to make the load feel lighter.

Clauses 1, 4, 10 and 11 of the UKCC Code of Professional Conduct refer to the individual practitioner's accountability in this area. The latter two are particularly relevant to the idea of identifying and dealing with major stressors.

Clause 10 reads:

> Have regard to the environment of care and its physical, psychological and social effects on patients/clients, and also to the adequacy of resources, and make known to appropriate persons or authorities any circumstances which could place patients/clients in jeopardy or which militate against safe standards of practice.

I can remember, as a first year nursing student, protesting at the treatment of an elderly woman of poor sight and hearing who, while recovering from hip surgery, often felt sick and occasionally vomited. A barium meal was ordered and the woman was thrown on to a trolley and forced to endure indignities (being shouted at, roughly handled, and left in a draughty corridor with only me to help her) at the hands of a very senior consultant radiologist. While the investigation was being carried out she was pushed up on the X-ray table with sufficient force to rip the intravenous infusion from an already bruised and swollen arm. Barium was forced down her with only minimal explanation, and when I protested the radiologist swore and told me to 'mind my place' while the assisting radiographer quickly looked away.

When the woman was upset and thoroughly bewildered we were sent away and told to report back later that afternoon. On returning to the ward somewhat shaken myself I made the patient as comfortable as I could and asked to speak to the ward sister, who was fortunately very experienced and prepared to believe what I told her.

I was summoned to the matron (the then equivalent of director of nursing services) who thanked me for telling her, but asked whether I was aware that the consultant was the most senior in the faculty, and probably one of the world's most eminent? I really could not expect to pursue the matter if I wished to continue my training.

Strangely, it was decided that a repeat investigation was not required and I was allowed to go on caring for the patient throughout her stay. How it would have helped to have had Clause 10 to guide me, and the means by which to make my protest public. Even ten years ago the notion of the nurse as the patient's advocate had not been formally recognised, and the stress involved in being unable to act properly in the patient's defence was almost enough to persuade me to give up altogether. It was left to a clinical teacher to absorb this stress, and to persuade me that there was nothing to gain from 'abandoning the cause'.

Although the Code is the tool of the qualified practitioner it is still the model for all current nursing students in preparing for their roles as nurses and advocates of the patient.

Clause 11 acknowledges the effects of unacceptable pressures on the nursing team:

> Have regard to the workload and the pressures on professional colleagues and subordinates and take appropriate action if these are seen to be such as to constitute abuse of the individual practitioner and/or to jeopardise safe standards of practice.

Stress signals can manifest themselves in different ways according to the individual's predisposition and personality. An increased awareness of potential stressors brought about by better education and an understanding of individual and group responses to it can help to prevent stress from becoming unmanageable and overwhelming.

Stress reducing strategies

The special stressors applicable to returning nurses and health visitors could include:

● Initial nervousness and insecurity when faced with unfamiliar surroundings and situations.
● Not wishing to appear stupid or ill-informed in front of patients and colleagues.
● Lack of up to date knowledge leading to a potential crisis of confidence.
● Apprehension at potential mistakes.
● Meeting new people.
● High and unrealistic expectations of the re-entry programme or proposed job.

- Concern over the changes in lifestyle to undertake the job.
- Awareness that others often younger and less experienced will be in a position of authority at work.

Recognition from educators and managers that such stress exists and is legitimate is a very important initial strategy in coming to terms with both the positive and the negative influences of stress.

Tackling an inherent lack of confidence in the stressed individual is also crucial (as discussed in chapter 2), as is increasing the individual's awareness that they are not alone, and that networks can be developed to reduce its impact.

The use of assertiveness and relaxation skills heighten the sense of self-worth, as do peer support groups and reliable and empathetic mentor systems.

Nash[15] describes the use of 'stress skills' in combating the stress that works against us, and in putting the same stress to work for us instead. She describes 'discernment' – 'the ability to recognise and acknowledge particular strands in a situation' – as underlying all stress skills:

> Many situations of stress feel like a tangled knot of coloured threads – the more you pull at it the worse it gets. But if the different strands can be gradually disentangled, the situation becomes easier. It depends as much on the recognition and discernment of each strand as the ability to follow it through.

Her strategies include acknowledging you own sense of wholeness, of taking care to listen properly, to take charge of whatever choice you make; to rechannel blame and guilt into something more positive, and to make space and time for what is really important, for instance not finding yourself bogged down in trivia when there are more important issues to be confronted.

Nash's approach of wholeness is primarily a Christian outlook on stress which provides an interesting contrast to Meg Bond's major work on stress in nursing entitled *Stress and Self Awareness*.[16] I would strongly recommend both books in providing enlightening routes out of a very demanding and difficult area.

The transition from returner to returned can be helped by the understanding of colleagues and tutors, but inevitably your success in meeting any new demands made upon you will depend on your own reserves of willpower, assertiveness, give and take, and common sense.

Effective coping strategies have to confront stressors directly; hoping that they will go away or get better is not usually enough. You will gradually learn to decode the complex messages which differentiate between acceptable, manageable, positive stressors which can be successfully modified, and those which require additional outside help to be contained.

Take some time to read around the subject of stress, and to experiment with new ways of coping. The further reading I recommend can help you to challenge some commonly held assumptions about where stress comes from, and should help you to structure your own plan for coping with it in a way which is appropriate to you personally.

References

1.   T. Clay, *Nurses, Power and Politics* (London: Heinemann, 1987).
2.   D. Owen, *Our NHS* (London: Pan, 1988).
3.   UKCC, *Government Approval in Principle* (press release) (London: UKCC, 1988).
4.   UKCC, *Project 2000 – A New Preparation for Practice* (London: UKCC, 1986).
5.   A. Emerton, *Chair's address to Council*, 16 January (London: UKCC, 1987).
6.   UKCC, *The Facts about Project 2000* (advisory document) (London: UKCC, 1988).
7.   UKCC, *The Enrolled Nurse and Preparation for Entry to a First Level Part of the Register* (Document PS & D/88/05, (London: UKCC, 1988).
8.   UKCC, *The Code of Professional Conduct for the Nurse, Midwife and Health Visitor*, 2nd edn (London: UKCC, 1984).
9.   The Nurses', Midwives' and Health Visitor's Act, 1979, Section 2(5).
10. R. H. Pyne, 'On being accountable', *Health Visitor*, **61** (1988) pp. 173–5.
11. P. Burnard and C. M. Chapman, *Professional and Ethical Issues in Nursing – the Code of Professional Conduct* (Chichester: John Wiley & Sons, 1988).

12. R. H. Pyne, 'The UKCC code of conduct', *Nursing*, **3** (1987) pp. 510–12.
13. M. Bamber, 'Slant on stress', *Nursing Times*, Nursing practice supplement, **84**, No. 11 (1988).
14. J. Salvage, *The Politics of Nursing* (London: Heinemann, 1986).
15. W. Nash, *At Ease With Stress* (London: Darton, Longman & Todd, 1988).
16. M. Bond, *Stress and Self-Awareness* (London: Heinemann, 1985).

Recommended reading

Project 2000

L. Swaffield, 'The new face of nursing?', *Nursing Times*, **84**, No. 31 (3 August, 1988).
M. Brown, 'Better get ready: the implications of Project 2000 for ward staff as teachers', *Nursing Times*, **84**, No. 35 (31 August, 1988).

Accountability

P. Burnard and C. Chapman, '*Professional and Ethial Issues in Nursing – the Code of Professional Conduct*' (Chichester: John Wiley & Sons, 1988).
R. Pyne, 'On being accountable', *The Health Visitor*, June, **61**, No. 6 (June 1987).
K. Rea, 'Negligence', *Nursing*, **3**, No. 14 (February 1987) pp. 533–6.
R. Rowden, 'The UKCC code of conduct: accountability and implications', *Nursing*, **3**, No. 14 (February 1987) pp. 512–16.
J. Tingle, 'Nursing ethics and the law, including accountability and responsibility', *Senior Nurse*, **8**, No. 2 (February, 1988).
UKCC, *The Code of Professional Conduct for the Nurse, Midwife and Health Visitor*, 2nd edn (London: UKCC, 1984).

Advocacy

S. Porter, 'Siding with the system', *Nursing Times*, **84**, No. 41 (12 October 1988).
J. Sawyer, 'On behalf of the patient', *Nursing Times*, **84**, No. 41 (12 October 1988).
C. Webb, 'Speaking up for advocacy', *Nursing Times*, **83**, No. 34 (26 August 1987).

Professional standards

A. Kitson, 'Raising the standards, an introduction to assessment and quality assurance tools', *Nursing Times*, **84,** No. 25 (22 June 1988).

Enrolled nurses

P. Bradshaw, H. Brown and D. Moore, 'Ripe for conversion? Selection and curricula for conversion courses', *Senior Nurse*, **7,** No. 3 (September 1987).
'Conversion courses for enrolled nurses to become RGNs', *The Professional Nurse*, **4,** No. 1 (October 1988).
M. Cottingham, 'The long and winding road', *Nursing Times*, **84,** No. 7 (17 February 1988).
P. White and K. Karim, 'Converting the Faithful', *Nursing Standard* (17 September 1988).

Support workers

N. Dickson and A. Cole, 'Nurse's little helper?' *Nursing Times*, **83,** No. 10 (11 March 1986).
UKCC, *Position paper on the Development of the Support Worker Role* (London: UKCC, 1988).

Stress

For recommended reading on stress please see the separate bibliography given in chapter 7.

CHAPTER 6

Returning to Learning

'Where there is much desire to learn
there of necessity will be much arguing,
much writing,
many opinions: for opinion in good men
is but knowledge in the making'

John Milton, 1608–1674

If you can forgive Milton for what might now be considered to be a sexist remark, there is a 17th century solidity about his philosophy of learning. Strangely, it has taken the nursing education establishment in Britain until now to recognise the value of debate, and the need to educate nurses for their own sake, as well as in the interests of patient care.

The very evolution from the concept of nurse 'training' to nurse 'education' is a relatively recent development which has really only gained momentum in the past eight to ten years. The word 'training' implies a moulding, a conformity to a stereotype, and is applied more usually to technical apprenticeships where rote learning of facts, routines and technical data is essential to enable a trade to be carried out efficiently.

But where does this leave nursing? Is nursing purely a matter of imitating and repeating rote tasks, and therefore unworthy of anything more than the sympathetic application of a set of predetermined rules?

The exercise of accountability, and of professional judgement, by their very definitions require much more in-depth knowledge, and the ability to analyse and evaluate information, and to relate both to the care of individuals and to client groups. The ability to identify and assess problems, and to understand their effects and limitations on patients cannot be learned passively and by rote, if only because no two people respond to the same problem in exactly the same way.

If you have been away from nurse education for some time you will be very pleasantly surprised by the much more interactive and civilised approach to learning apparent in most schools and colleges of nursing. The example of our colleagues in the higher education sector has had a major, positive influence on the educational methods employed by nurse educators, even if the initial response to this has at times been guarded by the 'old school' establishment.

The move is much more towards learning by and from personal experience, not just in nursing, but from everyday life, from contact with others and from previous employment, anything which adds an extra dimension to the way we perceive problems and set about dealing with them. The didactic approach of preaching to 'learners' (rather than 'students') and of spoonfeeding them with preset values and objectives is gradually being replaced by a much more human approach where students are enabled to question and study, and to add to knowledge themselves as they extract the best from individual learning experiences.

The move towards student and supernumerary status for all those undertaking a nursing education – not just undergraduates – and the plans to replace training allowances with a non means tested grant, means that the position and role of the student is expected to shift dramatically from learning 'by trial and error' to learning from practical experience *and* knowledge based on authoritative research. Research skills are now taught very early in nurse education, so that the value of research is appreciated not as an ephemeral, ivory tower point of view, but as a solid foundation for basing nursing care on the most effective means currently available of providing care.

You might argue that the only way for a nurse to learn how to dress a wound or administer an injection is by observing and practising the skill until she is competent. Research does not argue with this, but it does cut out a lot of hard work by providing evidence on the best methods, treatments, or products available from which you can begin to make choices and evaluate the effectiveness of care given as a result.

Returning nurses can feel threatened by the mention of 'research based care' or 'experiential learning'. I believe that this may be due to the sense of security and feeling of being safe which comes from familiar methods and tasks.

The idea that the care you provide might be questioned or challenged is an entirely new experience for nurses 'trained' by traditional methods. It is refreshingly easy to overcome initial fears, however, if you are prepared to enter into the debate, and not allow yourself to take comments or criticisms personally when a student peers at you agog for carrying out what they see as an archaic approach.

More information on acquiring research skills is provided in the next chapter. As an introduction to refreshing reading and study skills, Philip Burnard, lecturer in the School of Nursing Studies at the University of Wales College of Medicine, describes what is meant by experiential and student centred learning. An example of a useful self assessment exercise is also provided.

Experiential learning

There is an increasing realisation that a need exists to bridge the 'theory-practice' gap in nursing. One way of achieving this is the means of using nurses' personal and life experience in the learning situation. Increasingly, 'experiential learning methods' are being used in nurse education, both in basic and postbasic programmes. In order to appreciate what experiential learning is, it may be helpful to consider three types of knowledge (Figure 6.1).

Theoretical knowledge is 'textbook' knowledge. It is knowledge that derives from scholarship and from research. Practical knowledge, on the other hand is knowledge about how to *do* things. Whenever a nurse gives an injection or changes a dressing she demonstrates the application of practical knowledge. Both of these types of knowledge have traditionally been included in nurse education programmes.

Experiential knowledge, however, is knowledge gained through direct experience with a person, place or thing. It is personal or private knowledge that develops out of familiarity

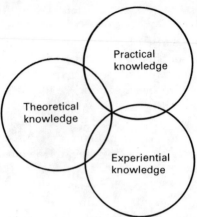

Figure 6.1
Three domains of knowledge

with a situation. For example, before a person visits America, they may have theoretical knowledge about it. When they visit the country, however, that knowledge is transformed – the person's knowledge of the place becomes altogether different. It becomes personal, rich and alive. This, then, is the nature of experiential knowledge. It derives from the process of living.

Nurses gain a valuable store of experiential knowledge through working with patients and colleagues in the wards and in the community. They also develop it through the process of living, itself.

Experiential learning methods aim to develop that domain of knowledge by offering a range of experience through which the nurse can learn. Examples of experiential learning methods include role play, structured group exercises and counselling skills exercises. They differ from more traditional educational techniques which focussed more on theoretical and practical knowledge. Experiential learning methods ask nurses to experience something for themselves. Thus the learning that follows is personal and yet highly meaningful to the individual.

Experiential learning methods are particularly useful as a means of developing interpersonal and communication skills. If, for instance, the nurse is to develop a range of counselling skills there seems little point in her learning it in a theoretical sense. Nor can she merely learn a mechanical set of techniques. What, perhaps, she needs to do is to learn to counsel by doing counselling and by being counselled.

The methods have other applications in nursing. Many practical nursing procedures from bedmaking to changing a dressing may best be learned through the nurse experiencing what these procedures feel like from the patient's point of view. Thus many nurse educators now set up simulations in the nurse education centre or the ward which allow direct experience of practical nursing skills.

Such direct experience helps the nurse to develop sensitivity and self-awareness. To experience something, ourselves, is to make us more sensitive to the needs and wants of others.

As we have seen, experiential learning methods may be encountered on a wide range of nurse education courses, including Back to Nursing courses. Table 6.1 offers examples of experiential learning activities used in nurse education.

Table 6.1
Examples of experiential learning activities used in nurse education

---

Role play
Brainstorming
Pairs exercises
Co-counselling activities
Structured group exercises
Relaxation exercises
Meditation
Role-rehearsal
Skills-rehearsal
Games
Simulation
Exercises involving reflection on the past
Gestalt exercises
Encounter group activities
Counselling exercises
Transactional analysis exercises
Management exercises
Guided fantasy
Problem-solving activities

Student-centred learning

One of the aims of modern nursing is to encourage patient autonomy. It is the patient who helps to decide on the course of his care and he may be asked to help to draw up objectives of care.

In keeping with this approach, educational methods in nurse education are increasingly moving towards a student-centred, negotiated approach to learning. In the past nurse educators decided on what and how learners should learn in the process of nursing. In recent years, however, has come the realisation that adults learn best when *they* have a say in what and how they learn. After all, not everyone learns in the same way. Some learn best from books, others from lectures and yet others from free and open discussion. Out of this diversity has emerged the notion of student-centred learning. In the student-centred approach, it is the *student* (or learner) who decides what and how she learns. Thus a course tutor may invite workshop members to identify their own learning needs, to write learning objectives and consider ways in which they would like to learn the new skills or information they need.

Such an approach takes into account different people's knowledge and skills levels, their varying educational, cultural and life experience. In the student-centred approach all this variety is used and incorporated into the learning process. Thus learning is no longer a passive activity involving the tutor 'filling' the learners with new ideas and facts. Instead, learning becomes an active, dynamic process that respects individual differences, needs and wants.

Many schools of nursing, colleges and university departments now use the student-centred approach in teaching nursing knowledge and skills. The approach is also frequently encountered on refresher courses. Table 6.2 illustrates how the approach may be applied in a back to nursing workshop.

Both the concepts of experiential learning and student-centred learning reflect the changing appreciation of the needs of the individual to develop and grow. We do not all live the same lives nor do we all need the same things. Experiential learning and student-centred learning can enable us to develop an increased awareness of helping people to make choices for

106

Table 6.2
Stages in the process of applying the student-centred approach in a
back to nursing workshop

Stage one	Negotiation with workshop members of learning objectives for the workshop
Stage two	Identification of learning resources within the group (including both workshop participants and facilitator)
Stage three	Planning of structure and content of workshop based on previous two stages
Stage four	Learning activities in line with plan
Stage five	Evaluation of learning with reference to stage one

themselves. If *we* can choose the means by which we learn nursing, we are more likely to allow others to choose the way they are cared for.

Both experiential learning and student-centred learning approaches are particularly suited to the adult learner. Adults bring a wealth of life experience to the learning situation and such experience can be a vital component in the educational encounter. Indeed, such life experience is, of course, a form of experiential knowledge, itself! All such knowledge must be of value in nursing, where a wide range of people from a broad range of cultures are cared for daily in a variety of contexts both at home and in the hospital setting.

Self-assessment

In order to plan further educational or skills programmes it is necessary, periodically, to stop and review progress. Self-assessment methods are useful, here, in that they can be carried out by the individual without the need of a tutor or teacher.

One simple self-assessment method is to draw up two columns: one lists recent achievements, the other further needs (Table 6.3). These two lists may then be used to identify further training needs and goals. The goals may be used as a personal memory-aid or discussed with a peer, tutor or nurse manager. The point of such an exercise is to clearly focus on present

Table 6.3
Simple self-assessment form

Self-Assessment: Name D. Jones	
Date: 18.4.88	
1 Learned new insulin measurements	1 Need more practice in giving subcutaneous injections
2 Learned ten new drug names and dosage	2 Need to brush up on medical condition
3 Read booklet on schizophrenia	3 Need to revise nursing care of mentally ill people

Goals
1 Practice giving a range of injections
2 Revise drugs and side effects
3 Obtain books on psychiatric nursing

learning needs and to clarify the process of learning.

Another method of self-assessment involves a friend or colleague. Here, the two people meet and each takes ten minutes to reflect on and verbalise the achievements that they have made and identify further needs. During this ten minutes, the other colleague merely listens to the other person's assessment. After the ten minute period, both people switch roles and the 'listener' becomes the one who reflects and verbalises.

Again, this method can be used to identify future learning goals. Its advantage is that it allows a far deeper and richer assessment to be made than the pen and paper exercise. It also serves as a useful means of relieving stress through review of recent weeks. Once established, the 20 minute process can be repeated at frequent intervals.

Self assessment may also take place in a group context. A small group of about five or six colleagues meet and each, in turn, reviews the past week in terms of achievements and future needs. Once each has had a turn, the group may spend a few minutes discussing possible methods of achieving any identified learning needs. Again, such a group, meeting on a regular basis, may serve as a stress-reducing medium. A problem shared, after all, is said to be a problem halved.

All these methods have been used in nurse education in recent years and reflect the student-centred approaches being adopted by many nurse educators.

Continuing your professional education

In its strategy for continuing education provision for qualified nurses in Scotland, the Scottish National Board for Nursing, Midwifery and Health Visiting accepts in principle the recommendations of a working party on continuing education and professional development for the three professions which reported in 1981. [1]

It is valuable to reiterate these recommendations as they very clearly convey the rationale behind current trends:

> There is a longstanding belief, in many walks of life, that basic preparation should suffice for a lifetime of practice. This belief is being challenged. Members of the nursing profession, who once assumed that training for registration would equip them for a career in nursing now realise that this is no longer the case. As with other professionals, they must learn and relearn throughout their professional lives if they are to keep pace with modern trends and changing needs.
>
> This awareness is relatively new, but if a nursing service of high quality is a goal to be achieved, nurses must have an understanding of human behaviour and the knowledge and skills to implement new technologies.
>
> Formal nursing courses reflect these concerns, but there is at present no mechanism for updating the knowledge of those who qualified some time ago. Experience does not necessarily fill this gap as people learn very differently from experience.
>
> In future, initial teaching must reflect the opinion that education in nursing, as in all professions, must continue after first qualification and opportunities are needed to make this a reality.

Scotland is ahead of the rest of the UK in providing an accessible modular system of continuing education whereby qualified nurses can undertake planned learning experiences in the form of 'modules' designed to meet the needs of different clinical specialties, and in more generic form, drawing from major areas of study drawn from moral, legal and political issues related to nursing, nursing practice, technology and science related to nursing.

Newly qualified nurses are expected to receive an orientation and induction programme appropriate to their appointments, followed by a consolidation period for a minimum period of three months, when it is recommended that a few hours each week be set aside for learning periods either with other newly qualified staff or as self-directed learning.

Following assessment and successful completion of a period of consolidation the nurse is then encouraged to proceed into a two part professional studies programme which leads to the National Board for Scotland Diploma in Professional Studies.[2]

Providing the resources and the opportunities to follow this example is a major consideration for the statutory and professional bodies throughout the UK. In an ideal world every qualified nurse would have the chance to further her professional education in this way.

The reality is of course very different, and although more initiatives are being introduced, much at present depends on the individual nurse's attitude towards continuing her education, and on her initiating the process for herself.

The boom in study days and conferences and in nursing literature is evidence of consumer demand for enjoyable ways of adding to professional knowledge, and there is now no need whatever to view continuing education as a chore and a duty to be carried out in isolation from colleagues and friends.

Many nursing studies departments have tutors with a specific remit for assisting nurses with their postbasic education, and they are usually very happy to provide assistance and advice to nurses currently in practice.

Examples of the many post-registration opportunities available are given in Jill Baker's book *What Next? Post-basic Opportunities for Nurses*[3] and in a book prepared by the Department of Health and the Central Office of Information entitled *Which way – continuing education for first level registered nurses,*[4] available from the careers centres addresses given in appendix 3.

Refreshing reading and study skills

The first thing you may find yourself doing in advance of this is blowing the dust from old textbooks in a fleeting fit of nostalgia. However thick the dust on your bookshelves may be you will either be reassured that you still remember a great deal of what you originally learnt from your training and former jobs, or you will be seized by momentary panic at how much you have forgotten.

The late 1980s have witnessed a virtual revolution in the range and quality of learning materials produced for nurses of every clinical specialism and professional interest. It is less usual to talk about nursing 'textbooks' as such. Reading is encouraged across the whole spectrum of nursing literature rather, reflecting in part the principles of holism; of caring for the whole person rather than being disease or disorder linked.

The materials you will be expected to use and enjoy will include a wide range of nursing journals, some of them well established and some which are entirely new to the market. The move to place nurse education within the realms of higher education has encouraged publishers to be more outward looking, and to provide more specialist in-depth titles, rather than vast tomes which promise to deliver comprehensive knowledge and yet which fail to do so by being too general. The books being published now are more attractive and relevant; they are usually written by experienced and practising nurses rather than doctors, and as a result are more appealing to the reader and are reviewed more enthusiastically than has been the case in the past.

Distance and open learning materials can be used effectively at home, obviating the need to have a tutor constantly at your elbow.

You will have more freedom to explore what interests you rather than being directed in your study by adherence to arbitrary book lists which encourage regurgitation of facts and diagrams without any analysis of the content.

Audio-visual materials, cassettes and videotapes, and access to computer based learning will simplify a lot of what used to be dull and repetitive work. By responding to your own learning needs rather than being expected to absorb blanket information as a group, you will be able to chart your own progress more accurately, develop and extend your interests and expertise, and research new materials as and when you feel the need.

111

You will probably appreciate some guidance and direction early on in your reading, and for this reason chapter 7 provides bibliographies which are intended to give you a flavour of current methods and ideas.

The skills required for proficient reading take time to acquire. I have been an avid reader since nursery school, and so find it very difficult to understand my headmaster husband when he dawdles over anything except travel brochures and restaurant menus! It does seem that some people would consider themselves natural and enthusiastic readers, while others need persuasion and encouragement to do anything other than 'dip' into a book.

You can begin by identifying different reading skills: skim or rapid reading, concentrated reading, information gathering, and reading which is done purely for pleasure and entertainment.

Skim-reading is fine if you are hoping only to get the 'gist' rather than the finer points of a piece, but dangerous if you are hoping to absorb information, or need to consider all sides of an argument. Silent, concentrated reading, however, needs time, space and peace and quiet, away from the demands of work, the family, your social life and television. It needs to be planned ahead rather than squeezed in around other commitments, particularly if you are preparing written work or you have to present a seminar.

It can be helpful to limit your reading time, allowing time for taking notes, or responding to queries. When you know you only have half an hour or so you can become quite absorbed and interested, and quite jealous of the limit you have set yourself. You can then congratulate yourself for going over your time, or at least by persevering satisfy yourself that you have made a little headway.

Library skills

It is a good idea to spend some time initially on familiarising yourself with your nursing library, and any specialist collections which may be of use to you. Librarians usually produce a guide to using their libraries. You can also make an appointment with the librarian or one of his staff so that the classification system can be explained to you together with any skills involved in scanning the microfiche for details of authors, articles and sources.

Returners often express difficulties in knowing where to begin, on which books to buy and which to borrow. Some course tutors supply their own introductory reading lists, and most specify 'musts' such as the UKCC Code of Professional Conduct; but others will arrange an early library session so that you are free to browse and survey what is available locally. This is unlikely to give you enough time to appreciate the breadth of materials on offer, however, and you could certainly supplement this by obtaining catalogues from nursing and medical book suppliers and by reading the book reviews in the nursing journals.

Both the RCN and HVA collections are impressive, and current bibliographies are available by subscription on application to the librarians. These are as comprehensive an update as you are likely to get in the UK. Both libraries operate a system of postal loans, provided postal charges are met by the borrower. Details are available on request from the librarian.

Writing skills

These are best acquired by regular practice, by reading, and by disciplining yourself to avoid unnecessary jargon, ambiguity and frills. There are several tips on note-taking and writing skills in an excellent book prepared by the Open University for prospective students called *Preparing to Study*,[5] and I strongly recommend it to anyone who lacks confidence in this area. It is available from book suppliers Eddington Hook, 406 Vale Road, Tonbridge, Kent TN9 1XR, and costs £2.95 plus 95p postage.

Preparing to Study also looks at learning via discussion and improving reading skills. It gives help on presenting your thoughts on paper and on getting the best out of libraries and the media to expand your knowledge and boost your confidence.

Writing and reporting skills are now much more sophisticated than even five years ago, and much more is expected of nurses and health visitors in completing documentation, preparing care plans and relating progress and evaluation reports, and in providing background reports for the information and assistance of other health professionals.

Time spent studying how others write can be helpful, although old habits can take some time to die, and some nurses who have difficulty in grasping new concepts can persist in applying old rules to new procedures, so do be warned. Recommended reading on this subject is offered at the end of this chapter, but any opportunity you have to practise writing skills, in a workshop or as part of a coursework exercise, is time well invested. Memory and retention skills can also be tested on each other, and you can be surprised by the misunderstandings which can result from not listening properly, or from being given inadequate or misleading information.

The skills involved in communicating information well are, I think, often underestimated, and could usefully be the subject for extensive practical workshops as part of a responsible continuing education programme.

Organising yourself

Of all study skills, perhaps the most elusive is the ability to organise and manage time effectively. This may be a matter for personal negotiation between yourself, your flatmates, friends, family and so on, and you may have to forego other pursuits for a while in order to establish a good study habit.

If you are conscientious at organising your notes and materials so that they can be referred to easily, then you will quickly be able to build up a personal library and reference system. If, like me, you tend to sit on mountains of paper, and rely on your memory to root out a reference, then you will need to be strong and discipline yourself to filing items away as soon as you have finished with them, either in folders or binders or in cabinet or box file, depending on the amount of space you have available.

If, also like me, you have a weakness for stockpiling past copies of nursing journals because you intend to catch up on such and such an article, then it is worth investing in some proper journal binders. These are relatively inexpensive and can help to restore order to superficial chaos. They are usually obtainable from publishers and can be purchased singly or in batches, depending on your personal requirements.

References

1. SHHD, *Continuing Education for the Nursing Profession in Scotland: a Report of a Working Party on Continuing Education and Professional Development for Nurses, Midwives and Health Visitors* (Edinburgh: Scottish Home and Health Department, 1981).
2. NBS, *Continuing Education for the Nursing Profession in Scotland* (Edinburgh: The National Board for Scotland, 1987).
3. J. Baker, *What Next: post-basic opportunities for nurses* (Basingstoke: Macmillan Education 1988).
4. DHSS, *Which Way? Continuing education for first level nurses* (London: HMSO, 1988).
5. *Preparing to Study* (Milton Keynes: Open University, 1979).

Recommended reading

S. Andrews, 'An expert in practice. What are the skills needed to be a nurse practitioner?', *Nursing Times*, **84**, No. 26 (1988).

P. Burnard, *Learning Human Skills: a Guide for Nurses* (London: Heinemann, 1985).

P. Burnard, 'Integrated self awareness: a holistic model', *Nurse Education Today*, **6** (1986) pp. 219–22.

P. Burnard, 'Building on Experience', *Senior Nurse*, **8**, No. 5 (1988).

S. Head, 'The new pioneers, the role of the nurse practitioner in the Accident and Emergency department', *Nursing Times*, **84**, No. 26 (1988).

P. Honey, 'You are what you learn': the process of learning', *Nursing Times*, **84**, No. 36 (1988).

L. Hopps, 'Road to Confidence: the move from learner to teacher, some tips for the nervous', *Nursing Times*, **84**, No. 34 (1988).

J. Isard, 'Open alternatives, management education for nurses', *Senior Nurse*, **8**, No. 4 (1988).

G. Markham, 'Special cases, a look at the developing role of clinical nurse specialists', *Nursing Times*, **84**, No. 26 (1988).

P. Moorbath, 'A guide to nursing research literature', *Senior Nurse*, **8**, No. 1 (1988).

C. R. Rogers, *Freedom to Learn for the Eighties* (Columbus, Ohio: Merrill, 1983).

UKCC, *UKCC's Proposed Rules for the Standard, Kind and Content of Future Pre-registration nursing education* (London: UKCC, 1988).

B. T. Waltho *et al.*, 'Contract-learning – a student's perspective', *Senior Name*, **7**, No. 6 (1987).

CHAPTER 7

Changes in Nursing Practice

Competencies and the nursing practitioner

By the time a nurse qualifies and becomes eligible for registration on the UKCC's Professional Register, she will have satisfied the competencies (relevant to her specialism) for the registered nurse as set down in Rule 18 of the Nurses, Midwives and Health Visitors Rules Approval Order 1983 S–I–1983 No 873.

As a returner, these are the skills in which you will be expected to be competent before being allowed to return to practice. There is, as yet, no system in operation which allows your competence to be assessed to a national standard, and it will be left to the discretion of your service manager, and course tutors if you have undertaken a back to nursing course, to decide whether you are ready to return, or what additional guidance or preparation you may need to bring you up to the required standard.

Re-entry programmes may include practical clinical assessments, but it is more usual to rely on reports from any supervised clinical allocations undertaken during a course, and any personal assessments carried out by continuing education tutors, your mentor, or senior nurse assessors working in the area where you will be working.

Competencies for first level nurses (parts 1, 3, 5, 8 of the Register)

First level nurses are expected to 'acquire the competencies required to':

- Advise on the promotion of health and the prevention of illness.
- Recognise situations that may be detrimental to the health and well-being of the individual.
- Carry out those activities involved when conducting the comprehensive assessment of a person's nursing requirements.
- Recognise the significance of observations made of a patient and use these to develop an initial nursing assessment.
- Devise a plan of nursing based on the assessment, with the co-operation of the patient, to the extent that this is possible, taking into account the medical prescription.
- Implement the planned programme of nursing care, and where appropriate, teach and coordinate other members of the caring team who may be responsible for implementing specific aspects of the nursing care.
- Review the effectiveness of the nursing care provided and where appropriate, initiate any action which may be required.
- Work in a team with other nurses and with medical and paramedical staff and social workers.
- Undertake the management of the care of a group of patients over a period of time and organise the appropriate support service.

All these competencies are related to the care of the particular type of patient with whom she is likely to come in contact when registered in that part of the Register for which the student intends to qualify.

Competencies for second level nurses (parts 2, 4, 6, 7 of the Register)

Second level nurses are expected to 'acquire the competencies required to':

- Assist in carrying out comprehensive observation of the patient and help in assessing his care requirements.
- Develop skills to enable her (the nurse), to assist in the implementation of nursing care under the direction of a first level nurse.

● Accept delegated nursing tasks.
● Work in a team with other nurses, and with medical and para-medical staff and social workers.

These competencies are related to the care of the particular type of patient with whom the nurse is likely to come in contact when registered in that part of the Register for which the student intends to qualify.

These competencies will be revised in proposed amendments to the current legislation in line with UKCC policy and the setting up of educational reforms introduced by Project 2000 (see chapter 5).

The most obvious change in nursing practice apparent to returners is the active involvement of patients and clients in their own care. The preparation of the 'new' nurse proposed by Project 2000 will reflect and build on this trend of helping people to initiate and promote healthy lifestyles.

While health visitors are presently considered to be the experts in health promotion, in future nurses of every clinical specialty will be expected to play an important role in health promotion, and in educating patients and colleagues towards self help in addition to getting the very best out of available health resources and expertise.

This promises to make nursing as a career much more dynamic and pro-active, although the nursing role in caring for the sick and those people limited by disability will continue and develop in response to the needs expressed by society.

Emphasis on caring for people in their own homes and in the communities in which they live means that more and more initiatives and nursing teams will become community based. Care provided in hospitals will therefore be more acute, with patients being discharged earlier to the care of primary health teams of general practitioners, district and specialist community nurses, practice nurses and health visitors.

Managing change

In order to help you obtain a broad background to recent philosophical and clinical developments in nursing, I have resisted the urge to present you with my own very limited definitions of changes which have occurred, and instead I have prepared exercises and suggested reading based on the criteria outlined by the UKCC on desired outcomes for successful completion of a re-entry programme.

It is not possible to cover all the professional and clinical issues in a book of this size, and in any case this would require the expertise of specialists in the field. Instead I have included those topics which were raised most consistently by returners as a potential source of worry or concern, culled from my own background research for learning materials aimed at returning nurses and health visitors.

Broadly speaking, these are:

● The impact of new technologies in nursing.
● Changes in nursing management and in the nursing hierarchy.
● Practical handling skills, and developments in equipment to assist mobility and promote independence.
● Skills required for safe drug administration and management.
● Issues regarding infection control, and in particular the transmission of HIV and hepatitis.
● Pain assessment and control, and the care of the terminally ill person and his family.
● Planning individualised nursing care based on nursing models and the nursing process.
● Emergency procedures for cardiopulmonary resuscitation (especially the nurse's role).
● The extended role of the nurse and its implications for returners.
● Clinical policies and procedures.
● Wound care and management.
● Research skills.
● The experience of stress and stress management.
● Guidance on measures to ensure a safe environment, and issues related to health and safety at work.

The following activities and exercises may be pursued individually or in groups, and may provide a framework for individual study leading to personal or group presentations in seminars or workshops, dependent on the resources available and the provisions made for personal study in the course curriculum or re-orientation programme.

PRACTICE INSIGHT 1

The impact of new technologies in nursing

What are the group's perceptions of new technologies in medicine, and how might these be expected to influence nursing care? Are there any developments which might be described as nursing technologies, and if so, how did they originate?

Practice check

Identify at least three examples of technologies which are unfamiliar to you, but which are used routinely in your clinical environment. What information and assistance is available to you in achieving competence in these?

Recommended reading

D. Allan, 'Making sense of infusion pumps', *Nursing Times*, **84,** No. 35 (31 August 1988).
S. Clements, 'And so to beds' (new technologies in beds and mattresses), *Community Outlook* (September 1987).
B. Koch and J. Rankin (eds), *Computers and their Applications in Nursing* (London: Harper & Row, 1987).
P. Lowe and L. Newman, 'Handle with care, technology in a nuclear medicine department', *Nursing Standard*, **2,** No. 52 (1 October 1988).
B. Michie, 'Making sense of total parenteral nutrition', *Nursing Times*, **84,** No. 20 (18 May 1988).
C. Milne, 'Information technology and nursing care', *Nursing Standard*, **2,** No. 51, (24 September 1988).
F. Pickersgill, 'Disposables – the case against re-use', *Nursing Times*, **84,** No. 44 (2 November 1988).
T. Smith, 'The Body Report', (seven part series on advances in health care and technologies), *Observer Magazine supplement* (1988).
M. Stephenson, 'The case for day surgery', *Nursing Times*, **84,** No. 4 (27 January 1988).
W. M. Tsang and G. Griffin, 'Blood glucose measurement', *Nursing Times*, **84,** No. 25 (22 June 1988).

PRACTICE INSIGHT 2

Changes in nursing management/the nursing hierarchy

The most recent influential review of NHS management – the Griffiths report – became the central issue in a major RCN campaign aimed at restoring the nursing voice in the management hierarchy. What were the report's recommendations?

Practice check

How are local nursing related resources managed in your clinical area/by your employer? What hierarchy are you expected to work under, and how does this influence the quality of care you give to patients?

Recommended reading

T. Clay, *Nurses – Power and Politics* (London: Heinemann, 1987).

R. Griffiths, *NHS Management Review* (London: DHSS, 1983).

R. Rowden, *Managing Nursing* (London: Baillière Tindall, 1984).

PRACTICE INSIGHT   3

Practical handling skills

Safe lifting and handling skills can help to restore mobility and to rehabilitate patients. The correct use of hoists and Ambulifts can also help nurses to avoid back injury. What are the current guidelines on safe lifting and handling?

Practice check

Are there any written policies or guidelines provided for use in your district/clinical area? Have you received up to date information and instruction on the use of safe handling techniques relevant to your clinical environment?

Recommended reading

Back Pain Association/RCN, *The handling of patients – a guide for nurses* (London: RCN, 1987).
I. Hill, *Towards safe lifting practice* (Clinical nursing practice – Recent Advances in Nursing series No. 14) (Edinburgh: Churchill Livingstone, 1986).
RCN, *Focus on Restraint – Guidelines on the use of restraint in the care of elderly people* (London: RCN, 1987).

PRACTICE INSIGHT 4

Skills required for safe drug administration and management

Nursing responsibilities in this area vary widely according to specialisms and medical interventions. What are your responsibilities in this area likely to involve, and are you aware of the current legislation relating to nurses?

Practice check

What are your main worries regarding drugs? Are you confident regarding routes of administration, drug calculations, drug storage and possible side effects of drugs unfamiliar to you?

Recommended reading

M. Aslam, T. Friedman and A. Pollard, 'Wonder drugs: the administration of psychotropic drugs', *Nursing Times*, **84**, No. 30 (27 July 1988).

M. Burton, 'Drug update: the insulins', *The Professional Nurse*, **3**, No. 9 (1988).

M. Burton, 'Handling cytotoxic drugs', *The Professional Nurse*, **3**, No. 12 (1988).

G. Downie, J. Mackenzie and A. Williams, *Drug Management for Nurses* (Edinburgh: Churchill Livingstone, 1987).

D. Gould, 'Called to account: responsibilities of the clinical nurse', *Nursing Times*, **84**, No. 12 (23 March 1988).

J. Hecker, 'Improved technique in intravenous therapy', *Nursing Times*, **84**, No. 34 (24 August 1988).

M. Johnston, M. Fitzgerald and I. Hoffman, 'Drug-giving for enrolled nurses', *Nursing Times*, **84**, No. 2 (13 January 1988).

RCN Dept. of Nursing Policy and Practice, 'Drug Administration – a nursing responsibility' (London: RCN, 1987).

UKCC, *Administration of Medicines: A framework to assist individual professional judgement and the development of local policies and guidelines* (London: UKCC).

PRACTICE INSIGHT 5

Infection control

Many district health authorities now employ infection control
nurses. Are you familiar with their role, and your own, in
assisting her in the implementation of local policies?

Practice check

Identify three areas in your clinical setting which have implications for the transmission of infection, and outline ways in
which this can be avoided.

Recommended reading

C. Campbell, 'Could do better, nurses attitudes towards the issue of
handwashing', *The Journal of Infection Control Nursing, Nursing Times*, **84**,
No. 22 (1 June 1988).
D. Gould, *Infection and Patient Care – A Guide for Nurses* (London:
Heinemann, 1987).
J. Stanford, 'Professional Care for people with HIV/AIDS', *The Pro-
fessional Nurse*, **4**, No. 2 (1988).
J. Stanford, 'AIDS – how do you react?', *The Professional Nurse*, **3**, No. 8
(1988).
UKCC, *AIDS and HIV infection*, PC 88/03 (London: UKCC 1988).
K. Ward, 'The Role of the infection control nurse', *Nursing*, **3**, No. 30
(1988).

PRACTICE INSIGHT 6

Pain assessment and control, and the care of the terminally ill patient

How does your past nursing experience measure up to present expectations of your role in these areas?

Practice check

What are the facilities and measurements used to assess pain in your care of patients? Do patients have access to a pain control clinic or specialist practitioner? What preparation and support do you expect to call upon when dealing with dying people and their families?

Recommended reading

C. Alderman, 'Controlling pain', *Nursing Standard*, **3**, No. 2 (8 October 1988).
B. Cook and S. Phillips, *Loss and Bereavement* (Croydon: Lisa Sainsbury Foundation Series, 1988).
J. Neuberger, *Caring for Dying People of Different Faiths* (Croydon: Lisa Sainsbury Foundation Series, 1987).
B. Sofaer, *Pain – a handbook for nurses* (London: Harper & Row, 1984).
J. Trevelyan, 'Prevailing over pain': the work of a clinic which teaches psychological management of pain, *Nursing Times*, **84**, No. 33 (17 August 1988).
S. Wright, 'Why use measurement? Measuring pain' (adapted from *Measurement in Nursing*, an Open Learning Package produced by the Continuing Nurse Education Programme, Barnet College, London), *Nursing Times*, **84**, No. 4 (27 January 1988).

PRACTICE INSIGHT 7

Individualised nursing care based on nursing models and the nursing process

How does individualised nursing care differ from the care you have given in your earlier career as a nurse? How can nursing models be defined and in what ways do they support the process of nursing?

Practice check

What are the stages of the nursing process, and how has it evolved in patient care since its introduction to Britain from the United States in the 70s?

Recommended reading

P. Aggleton and H. Chalmers, *Nursing Models and the Nursing Process* (Basingstoke: Macmillan Education/Nursing Times, 1986).
J. M. Hunt and D. J. Marks-Maran, *Nursing Care Plans – the Nursing Process at Work, 2nd edn* (Chichester: John Wiley & Sons, 1986).
K. Luker, 'Do models work? The practical value and use of models in community nursing', *Nursing Times*, **84,** No. 5 (3 February 1988).
R. McMahon, 'Who's afraid of nursing care plans?', *Nursing Times*, **84,** No. 29 (20 July 1988).
N. Roper, W. Logan and A. Tierney, *The Elements of Nursing, 2nd edn* (Edinburgh: Churchill Livingstone, 1985).
V. Sowton, 'Carry Out Care Plans: improving communication between community and hospital', Tissue Viability supplement, *Nursing Times*, **84,** No. 13 (30 March 1988).
K. Ward, 'Not just the patient in bed 3, the use of bedside care plans', *Nursing Times*, **84,** No. 28 (13 July 1988).

PRACTICE INSIGHT   8

Emergency procedures for cardiopulmonary resuscitation

What provision exists to enable you to update this skill in line with current recommendations? Do you consider yourself proficient, and if not, why not?

Practice check

What are the policies regarding CPR in your clinical area, and who lays down the criteria for exempting particular patients from CPR?

Recommended reading

D. Allan, 'Making sense of ECGs', *Nursing Times*, **84**, No. 38 (21 September 1988).
T. R. Evans (ed.), *ABC of resuscitation* (reprints of articles on aspects of resuscitation, including ethics and advanced life support) (London: British Medical Journal, on behalf of the Resuscitation Council, 1986).
R. Goodwin, 'Cardiopulmonary resuscitation', Critical Care supplement on teaching CPR, *Nursing Times*, **84**, No. 34 (24 August 1988).
M. Sloman, 'Paediatric cardiopulmonary resuscitation', *Nursing Times*, **84**, No. 43 (26 October 1988).

Bibliographies

The extended role of the nurse

RCN and BMA, *The Duties and Position of the Nurse* (joint statement) (London: RCN, 1978).

R. Rowden, 'The extended role of the nurse', *Nursing*, **3**, No. 14 (1987) pp. 516–18.

Clinical policies and procedures

E. M. Jamieson, J. B. McCall and R. Blythe, *Guidelines for Clinical Nursing Practice* (Edinburgh: Churchill Livingstone, 1980).

P. Pritchard and J. David (eds), *The Royal Marsden Hospital Manual of Clinical Nursing Procedures*, 2nd edn (London: Harper & Row, 1988).

Health and safety

HVA, *Health and Safety in the Community* (London: HVA, 1984).

R. Rogers and J. Salvage, *Nurses at risk – A Guide to Health and Safety at Work* (London: Heinemann, 1988).

Wound care and management

S. Bale and K. Harding, 'Wound management', *Nursing Standard* (16 April 1988).

J. A. David, *Wound Management* (London: Martin Dunitz Ltd, 1986).

A. Ferguson, 'Best performer: a review of products available for effective wound care', *Nursing Times*, **84**, No. 14 (6 April 1988).

N. Harrild, 'A stitch in time', *Nursing Standard* (19 March 1988).

A. Johnson, 'Wound healing under the microscope', *Community Outlook* (January 1987).

A. Johnson, 'Modern wound care products', *The Professional Nurse*, **3**, No. 10 (1988) pp. 392–8.

J. Roberts, 'Penny wise–pound foolish', *The Journal of Infection Control Nursing, Nursing Times*, **83**, No. 37 (16 September 1987).

S. Thomas, 'Cost effective dressings', *Community Outlook* (September, 1988).

Research skills

R. Bergman, 'Research in community nursing', *Recent Advances in Nursing*, **15** (1987) pp. 27–51.

E. Clark, 'Research and common sense', *The Professional Nurse*, **3**, No. 9 (1988) pp. 344–8.

D. F. S. Cormack, *The Research Process in Nursing* (Oxford: Blackwell Scientific Publications, 1984).

J. Macleod Clark and L. Hockey, *'Research for Nursing – A Guide for the Enquiring Nurse'* (London: HM & M Publishers, 1981).

M. Moody, 'Illuminating research', Tissue Viability supplement, *Nursing Times*, **83**, No. 39 (30 September 1987).

Stress in nursing

P. Burnard, 'Coping with emotion in ICU nursing', *Intensive Care Nursing*, **3** (1987) pp. 157–9.

P. Burnard, 'No need to hide', *Nursing Times*, **84**, No. 24 (1988).

Distance Learning Centre, *Stress in Nursing*, Managing Care programme, Part 16 (London The Distance Learning Centre, 1988).

A. Faulkner and P. Maguire, 'The need for support', *Nursing*, **3**, No. 28 (1988).

C. Gillespie, 'Stress reducing strategies', *Nursing Times*, **83**, No. 39 (30 September 1987).

S. Goodwin, 'Stress in health visiting', *Recent Advances in Nursing*, **15**, (1987) pp. 99–111.

P. Maguire, 'Barriers to the psychological care of the dying', *British Medical Journal*, **291** (1985) p. 711.

R. G. Mitchell, 'The emotional cost of nursing', *Nursing*, **3**, No. 28 (1988).

R. H. Pyne, 'Confronting stress', *Nursing Times*, **83**, No. 27 (8 July 1987).

L. Swaffield, 'Sharing the load', *Nursing Times*, **43**, No. 36 (September 1988).

M. West and J. Savage, 'Visitations of distress', *Nursing Times*, **84**, No. 31 (1988).

Changes in health visiting practice

The HVA publish a recommended re-entry reading list, available from the Education Officer, The Health Visitor's Association, 50 Southwark Street, London SE1 1UN.

DHSS, *Neighbourhood Nursing – A focus for care*, the report of the community nursing review (England), otherwise known as the Cumberlege Report (London: HMSO, 1986).

HVA, *The Health Visitor's Role in Child Health Surveillance* (London: HVA, 1985).

HVA, *Health Visiting and School Nursing Reviewed* (London: HVA, 1987).

HVA, *Griffiths and After: the management of health visiting and school nursing* (London: HVA, 1987).

HVA, *All for Health: perspectives on education and training of health visitors* (London: HVA, 1987).

HVA, *Aspects of Child Abuse* (London: HVA, 1987).

HVA, *'Drug Misuse – Guidance for Health Visitors and School Nurses* (London: HVA, 1987).

K. Luker, *Evaluating Health Visiting Practice* (London: RCN, 1982).

W. Nash, M. Thruston and M. E. Baly, *Health at School* (London: Heinemann, 1985).

J. Orr, *Health Visiting* (Oxford: Blackwell Scientific Publications, 1985).

M. Piggott, 'Making the numbers add up', *Nursing Times*, **84**, No. 1 (6 January 1988).

P. Townsend and N. Davidson, *The Black Report* and M. Whitehead *The Health Divide*, now published as a single volume (London: Penguin Books, 1988).

Postscript

A study of the proposals for the new curriculum outlined in a consultation document issued by the UKCC in late 1988 has impressed upon me the revolution about to be experienced in nursing education, and made me wish wholeheartedly that I could begin my nursing preparation all over again.

Although plans for the curriculum will be debated and wrestled over until a suitable formula is agreed, there is no doubt that those fortunate enough to enter nursing in the 1990s will have a much more stimulating and intellectually demanding course ahead of them than any of my own contemporaries.

The plan and the hope is that initiatives for assisting nurses back into practice in the future will take their lead from this initial Project 2000 prototype preparation. If so, then the returning nurses and health visitors of the 90s can expect a very rewarding and enjoyable welcome back to nursing.

Appendix 1

THE UKCC CODE OF PROFESSIONAL CONDUCT FOR THE
NURSE, MIDWIFE AND HEALTH VISITOR

Each registered nurse, midwife and health visitor shall act, at
all times, in such a manner as to justify public trust and
confidence, to uphold and enhance the good standing and
reputation of the profession, to serve the interests of society,
and above all to safeguard the interests of individual patients
and clients.

Each registered nurse, midwife and health visitor is accountable for his or her practice, and, in the exercise of professional
accountability shall:

1   Act always in such a way as to promote and safeguard the
    well being and interests of patients/clients.

2   Ensure that no action or omission on his/her part or within
    his/her sphere of influence is detrimental to the condition
    or safety of patients/clients.

3   Take every reasonable opportunity to maintain and im-
    prove professional knowledge and competence.

4   Acknowledge any limitations of competence and refuse in
    such cases to accept delegated functions without first hav-
    ing received instruction in regard to those functions and
    having been assessed as competent.

5   Work in a collaborative and co-operative manner with other
    health care professionals and recognise and respect their
    particular contributions within the health care team.

6   Take account of the customs, values and spiritual beliefs of
    patients/clients.

7   Make known to an appropriate person or authority any conscientious objection which may be relevant to professional practice.

8   Avoid any abuse of the privileged relationship which exists with patients/clients and of the privileged access allowed to their property, residence or workplace.

9   Respect confidential information obtained in the course of professional practice and refrain from disclosing such information without the consent of the patient/client, or a person entitled to act on his/her behalf, except where disclosure is required by law or by the order of a court or is necessary in the public interest.

10   Have regard to the environment of care and its physical, psychological and social effects on patients/clients, and also to the adequacy of resources, and make known to appropriate persons or authorities any circumstances which could place patients/clients in jeopardy or which militate against safe standards of practice.

11   Have regard to the workload of and the pressures on professional colleagues and subordinates and take appropriate action if these are seen to be such as to constitute abuse of the individual practitioner and/or to jeopardise safe standards of practice.

12   In the context of the individual's own knowledge, experience, and sphere of authority, assist peers and subordinates to develop professional competence in accordance with their needs.

13   Refuse to accept any gift, favour or hospitality which might be interpreted as seeking to exert undue influence to obtain preferential consideration.

14   Avoid the use of professional qualifications in the promotion of commercial products in order not to compromise the independence of professional judgement on which patients/clients rely.

(*Second edition, November 1984*)

Appendix 2

NURSING JOURNALS AVAILABLE FROM HIGH STREET NEWSAGENTS

An extensive bibliography and list of periodical holdings is available on request from the RCN librarian. Your local nursing library should also be able to obtain a list of journals for you to which you can subscribe if you wish.

Weeklies

Nursing Standard, published by Scutari Projects Ltd, the publishing company of the Royal College of Nursing. Editor: Norah Casey. Editorial address: *Nursing Standard*, Viking House, 17–19 Peterborough Road, Harrow, Middlesex HA1 2AX. Telephone: 01–423 1066. Subscriptions: Subscriptions Department, Freepost, Harrow HA1 2BR.

Nursing Times (including *Nursing Mirror* following a merger in 1985), published by Macmillan Magazines Ltd. Editor: Linda Davidson. Editorial address: *Nursing Times*, 4 Little Essex Street, London WC2R 3LF. Telephone 01–379 0970. Subscriptions: PO Box 500, Leicester LE99 0AA.

Monthlies

The Professional Nurse, published by Austen Cornish, Editor: Elizabeth M. Horne. Editorial address: *The Professional Nurse*, Austen Cornish House, Walham Grove, London SW6 1QW. Telephone 01–381 6301. Subscriptions: Subscription Manager, Austen Cornish House, Walham Grove, London SW6 1QW.

Nursing (The Journal of Clinical Practice), published by Mark Allen Publishing Ltd. Editor: Cate Campbell. Editorial address: 24 Augustus Close, Brentford Dock, Brentford, Middlesex TW8 8QF. Telephone: 01–568 1556. Subscriptions: Sue Duffin, *Nursing* Subscription Department, Esco Business Services, Robjohn's Farm, Vicarage Road, Finchingfield, Essex.

Appendix 3

CAREERS INFORMATION ADDRESSES

England

ENB Careers Information Centre,
PO Box 356,
Sheffield S8 0SJ

Scotland

The Nursing Adviser,
Scottish Health Service Centre,
Crewe Road South,
Edinburgh EH4 2LF

Northern Ireland

The Recruitment Officer,
National Board for Northern Ireland,
RAC House,
79 Chichester Street,
Belfast BT1 4JR

Wales

The Chief Nursing Officer,
Welsh Office,
Cathays Park,
Cardiff CF1 3NQ

REDHILL MULTIDISCIPLINARY LIBRARY
REDHILL HOSPITAL
EARLSWOOD COMMON
REDHILL, SURREY.

Index

(Main entries appear in **bold** type)

Abroad
  nursing 16
Accommodation
  NHS rented **40**
Accountability ix, 6, **90–2**, 94, 99
Agency nursing **74–8**
Approval
  current re-entry programmes
    52, **56–7**
  training institutions 84
Assessments
  clinical 117
  motivation 9
  self motivation **107–9**

Back to nursing courses
  generally 4
  course content **64–6**
  course supervision **57**
  experiential learning and 107
  for health visitors **67–9**
  UKCC criteria and 50
  see also Re-entry programmes
Banks
  nursing **74–5**
Bibliographies 130–2
Books 4, 111

Care plans/planning 118, **128**
Career break 1
Career development/goals **5–17**
Career structure **7–8**
Careers advice agencies,
    Appendix 3
Change
  in health visiting practice 31–2
  in nursing management 123
  in nursing practice **117**
  managing 119–21
Childcare **44–7**

Clinical grading
  and returners **28–9**
  exercise 27
Clinical policies/procedures 130
Code of Professional Conduct
  (UKCC) 6, 7, 12, 21–3, 65,
    90–2, 94, 96, Appendix 1
Common Foundation Programme
  87
Competencies
  for first and second level
    nurses **117–19**
Consultation documents
  UKCC 51
Continuing education
  general background to **109–11**
  tutors 5, 60
Contracts of employment **28**, 39,
  77
Conversion courses
  to first level nursing 88–9
  UKCC policy and 88–9

Degrees
  in nursing and related social/
    life sciences 87
Dependents
  care of **41–7**
Desired outcomes
  UKCC criteria 66
Drug administration 125

Enrolled nurses
  recommended reading for 100
  the position of **88–90**
Experiential learning **103–8**
Extended role of the nurse 130

Funding
  re-entry programmes 52

pay awards 27

Grading *see* Clinical grading
Griffiths Report 1983 **14**, 123
Guidelines for Good Practice
    (UKCC) 2, **50–3**

Handling skills 124
Health and safety at work 130
Health visitors
    conditions of work 30–1
    indemnity insurance 30
    jobsharing 31
    new titles 55
    re-entry programmes for 67–9
    re-licensing and 55
Health Visitor's Association
    address 68
    general secretary viii
    residential courses 67–9
HIV and infection control 126
Hours of work 37–8

Indemnity insurance 17, 30, **60**
Independent sector
    employment 15–17, 78–9
Infection control 126
Interviews
    for courses/jobs 79

Job
    applications 79
    centres 73
    decisions 3
    description 23–5
    expectations **25–8**
    fairs and forums 70–3
    opportunities **10–16**
    sharing 30, 37
Journals
    nursing 111, **136–7**
    see also Library skills

Law and re-entry programmes 50
Learning needs 20–1, 63–4
Library skills **112–13**

Management

NHS **13–14**, 123
Managers'
    expectations 11
    obligations 22
Mandatory refreshment **50–3**
Manpower estimates 53

National boards 55–8, 63, **83–5**
Negligence 60
Neighbourhood nursing 132
New technologies 122
New titles 55–6
Nursing
    as a profession 5, 26–7
    competencies **117–19**
    models 128
    process 128
    skills 11–15, 19–21
    students 33

Pain assessment and control 127
Parttime work 38
Pay awards 27
Periodic fees
    and relicensing 53–5
    linked to re-entry 55
Politics
    NHS 81–2
Professional conduct *see* Code of
    committees 84–5
    functions 84–5
Professional standards **90–2**, 100
Project 2000 83, **85–7**, 99
Public sector employment 15–17

Reading skills 112
Recruitment
    campaign 49
    drives 71
    problems 49–50
Re-entry
    guidelines 50
    programmes **50–69**
    routes of 58–60, 70
    schemes 50
    see also Back to nursing courses
Registration status/update 54
Research

awareness   33
skills   14, 131
Respite care   43–4
Rules
  as in Nurses, Midwives and
    Health Visitor's Act,
    1979   65, 117

Safety at work   130
Self
  assessment   108
  help   23–5
Single Professional Register
  (UKCC)   53, 55, **56**
Specialisms in nursing   14–15
Statutory framework for the
  professions   83–5

Stress
  reading list   131
  reducing strategies   96–9
  the nature of   92–6

Transport
  to and from work   39

United Kingdom Central Council
  for Nursing, Midwifery and
  Health Visiting, (UKCC)   1,
  83–5

Wound care and management
  130
Writing skills   113–14